MEDICINE'S
NEW VISION

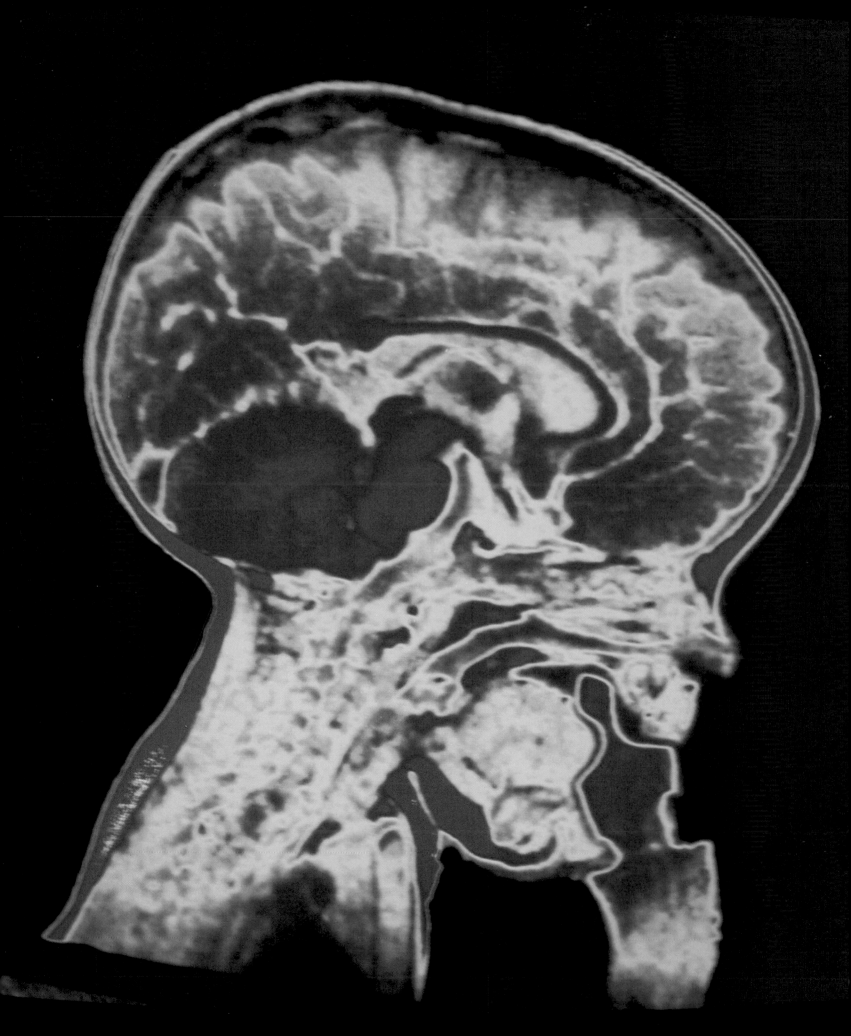

MEDICINE'S
NEW VISION

Howard Sochurek

Mack Publishing Company

Easton, Pennsylvania

Printed in the United States of America

Printer: Mack Printing Company,
        Easton, Pennsylvania

Designer: Anne M. Rhymer

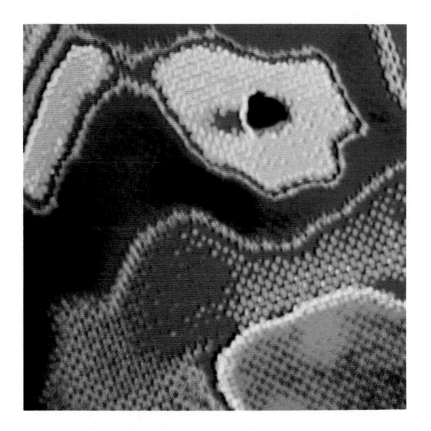

"... for with hidden diseases it is not as with the recognizing of colors: in colors one sees well what is black, green, blue, etc. But if there were a curtain before them, thou also wouldst not know. To see through a curtain requires effort where there has been none before."

Paracelsus (1493–1541) from *Seven Defensiones*

CONTENTS

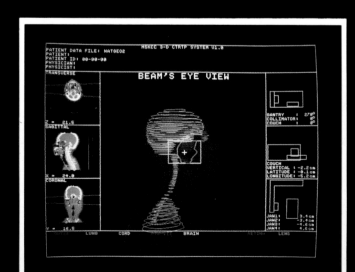

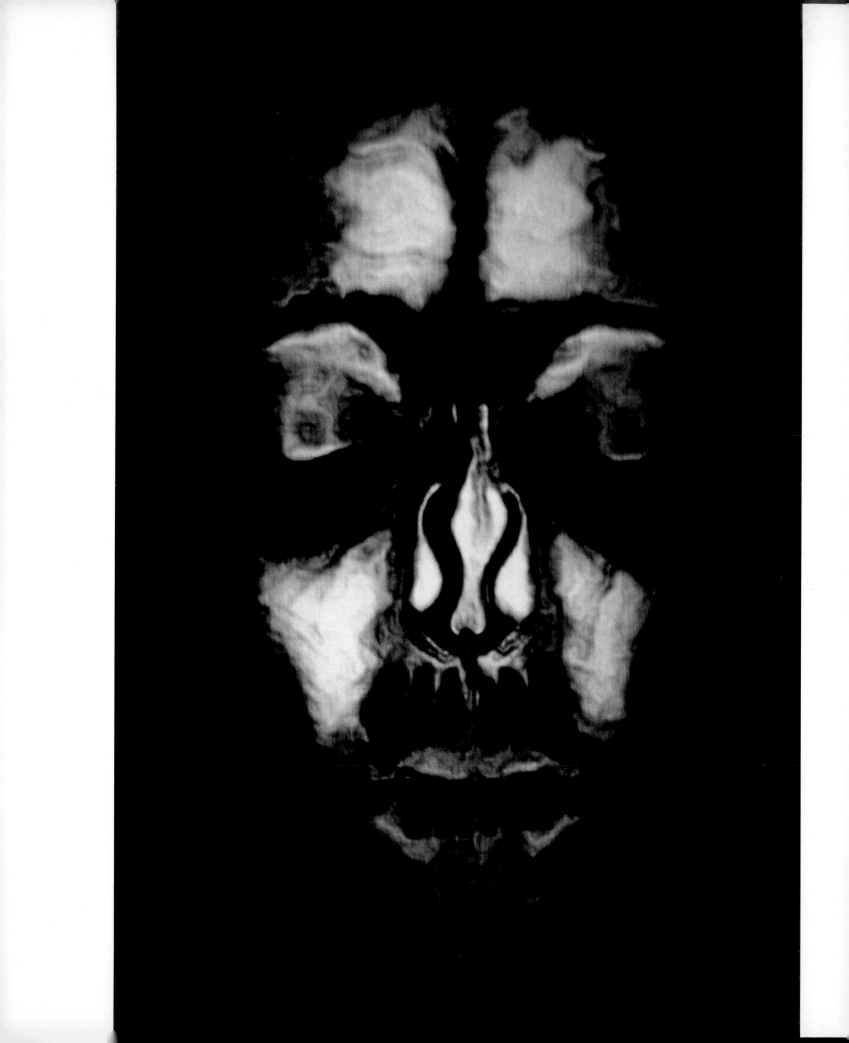

Foreword

The book in hand emphasizes the place of radiology in the medical scheme of things and underscores the radiologist's important role in medical diagnosis. The aim has been to convey this information using terms and pictures that the lay reader can understand. Members of the professional radiologic community will, we trust, view the book in this spirit and recognize that the public's need to know took precedence over encyclopedic portrayal of their fascinating—but often recondite—field of medical endeavor.

Similarly, hundreds of radiologists and allied scientists have made substantial clinical and technologic contributions to medical imaging in the nearly 100 years since Dr. Roentgen discovered the x ray, and their efforts have affected and continue to affect the quality of all our lives. Only a few are mentioned in the nine chapters that follow; a chronicle of radiologic achievers and achievements, however, would have blurred the author's focus and thwarted his mission.

To the reader of this book we offer the following advice: take time to learn about medical breakthroughs and advances, talk with and query your physician about all aspects of your treatment, find out what the medical risks and options are, read more books like the one you are holding. Your health is the most precious commodity you have.

The Board of Directors of the Radiological Society of North America expresses its gratitude to the author and publisher for bringing *Medicine's New Vision* into the light.

E. Robert Heitzman, M.D., Chairman
Malcolm D. Jones, M.D., President
Robert E. Campbell, M.D.
Carl J. Zylak, M.D.
Robert G. Parker, M.D.
Thomas S. Harle, M.D.
O. Wayne Houser, M.D.
Helen C. Redman, M.D.

Author's Introduction

In the Fall of 1985 I suggested an idea for a story to Bill Garrett, Editor of *National Geographic*, on the new breakthroughs in medical imaging. My plan was to explain the equipment, personally undergo radiologic tests, and offer real life accounts of persons that had been helped by the new imaging methods.

The assignment lasted about a year and took me from coast to coast and Europe as well. I interviewed hundreds of doctors and talked to scores of patients. The results of these efforts appeared in the January 1987 issue of *National Geographic* (cover and pages 1–40) under the title "Medicine's New Vision." Although I have been in journalism for 40 years, nothing that I had previously done met with the response I received from this story. Calls and letters came to me from all over the world asking for information and referral advice.

Representatives of the Radiological Society of North America—the largest educational association of radiologists and allied scientists in the world—came to see me shortly after the magazine appearance of "Medicine's New Vision." As a way to commemorate their 75th anniversary and raise public awareness about what radiologists do, they wondered whether the *National Geographic* piece could be expanded into a book that included the topics already covered plus several additional, more timely developments in the field, and that described more adequately the radiologist's role in medical diagnosis. With the encouragement and help of Tom Smith, Associate Editor of *National Geographic*, who permitted me to use the original work, I agreed to accept the assignment.

Another year of extensive travel and interviews has resulted in the work displayed on the following pages. I found that—more than any other medical specialist—the radiologist has harnessed the computer and devised technologies to extend his diagnostic abilities in exciting and innovative ways. Gathering this information has been a rewarding experience; I hope it will prove valuable to many more readers and patients.

Bronxville, New York
October 1, 1988

MEDICINE'S NEW VISION

763   0

Patient slides into MR tunnel.
Surface coil on knee gives greater
detail when imaging bone and soft
tissue. This machine is one of
medicine's new life savers.

I. MAGNETIC RESONANCE

"To see and be amazed"

To look into the inner depths of the body, to observe not only the details of anatomy but of function (physiology): that is both the promise and the reality of the revolutionary new diagnostic imaging technique called magnetic resonance (MR).

Made possible by computers which quickly process millions of bits of information, MR equipment consists of a tunnel-like magnet that sets up a magnetic field around the patient. This field causes the hydrogen atoms in the body to line up while a radio frequency signal is transmitted, in a brief burst, to upset the uniformity of the formation. When turned off, the hydrogen atoms (actually the protons in the atoms are imaged) return to their lineup and a small electric current is generated. By assessing and measuring the speed and volume with which the atoms return, the computer can display a diagnostic image on a monitor (TV screen). To get even more detail, surface coils can be placed on the body to receive the radio frequency pulses at an exact area of interest. And in a newer development, intravenous contrast materials can be introduced into the body to enhance image definition.

MR is revolutionary because it is noninvasive: no pain or radiation are involved. The procedure takes from 15 to 45 minutes depending on the number of views required. Views can be taken in cross section (axial), from front to back (coronal), or from side to side (sagittal).

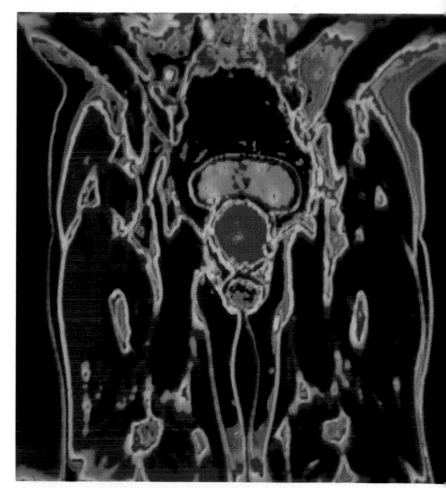

The prostate (center) glows red in this color-enhanced MR scan of the pelvis. Previously nearly impossible to image clearly, MR now does it painlessly and noninvasively.

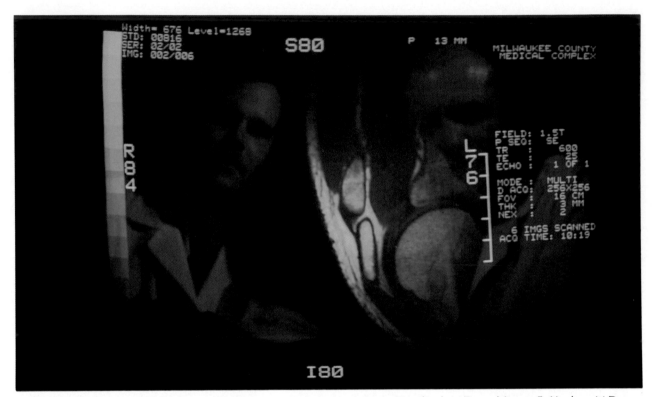

Radiologists J. Bruce Kneeland, M.D. and James E. Youker, M.D. are reflected in viewing station monitor of MR unit at the Medical College of Wisconsin. Shoulder structure of male patient is seen on the right of the screen. Text on tube refers to time, depth, area of coverage, and patient information.

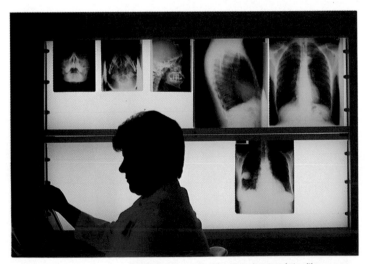

Radiologic technologist views plain film x-rays.

Traditional x-rays rely on variations of density on film. Because soft tissues produce little or no shadow, the ability of x-rays to delineate soft tissues is hampered in many cases. MR imagers, on the other hand, allow the radiologist to see soft tissues such as tumors in the brain and spinal column, fatty tissue, muscles, tendons, arteries, and details in the vertebrae and optic nerve—all with amazing clarity.

MR has witnessed an explosive growth in application. In 1982 only six machines were in operation in the United States. Today there are over 600 machines in operation, but many hospitals have patients waiting days to be scheduled for scans, with only emergency patients being taken care of immediately. Some hospitals, after a year's operation of a single machine, have ordered a second and third.

NO PAIN, NO STRAIN

Undergoing an MR exam is painless and easy. I had mine late one evening when the last regular patient had left the Long Island Diagnostic Imaging Center. Nancy Ryan, the receptionist, gave me a patient history form and a list of items that were forbidden in the scanning room. These included all surgical clips, credit cards, dentures and metallic implants.

The center's MR unit weighs 15 tons and is supercooled with liquid helium to minus 452° F. It cost $1,800,000 plus installation charges and incurs an $18,000 monthly bill for electricity and other costs. Ten patients a day undergo scanning which usually takes about 45 minutes per exam.

I left my shirt, tie, and trousers on but removed my watch, belt, and ring. "Why be scanned if there is nothing wrong with you?" asked Bill Seuffert, the technician at the console. "I wouldn't. They might find something," he said.

He had a point. At a major MR manufacturing and training center in Waukesha, Wisconsin, a young trainee who volunteered to be scanned was shocked to find that he had a huge brain tumor. He had been unaware of the tumor but had been troubled by occasional headaches. On inquiry, I found that a few of us may be living quite happily and normally with brain tumors that have little, if any, effect on our lives.

I lay down faceup on a sliding table, head slightly raised on a pillow-like bar, and was rolled into the magnet's tunnel which was 3' in diameter and 6' long. A red laser beam located the midline of my brain. Bill Seuffert, isolated from the magnet in the control room, communicated to me through an intercom. He asked if I was comfortable, told me to remain perfectly still, and said that he would do a cross-sectional (axial) scan of my midbrain.

For a minute or so, I heard what seemed to be the tapping of a hundred hammers—the clatter of magnetic coils as Bill set up the correct frequencies to achieve the best image definition.

A brief lull, and then the tapping of hammers began again—this time in earnest. As time passed within this magnetic field, 30,000 times stronger than the earth's, my skin tightened and I felt the older fillings in my teeth tingle.

The scan was completed in 2½ minutes. Had this been a full-scale search instead of a demonstration, there would have been an additional series of scans to provide the proper coronal and sagittal images and to obtain additional information for a particular area of interest.

After the scan, I got up from the table and walked to the control room. I felt just fine. Appearing on a black and white monitor, slowly emerging line by line, was the cross-sectional view of my brain. It showed no tumor or any other abnormalities. Clearly, MR is one of the safest and least traumatizing diagnostic tools available today.

THE EARLY DAYS AND BEYOND

The first MR imaging technique is attributable to Paul Lauterbur when, in 1972, he was able to generate the first two-dimensional image of proton density. Other pioneering work was done at Nottingham University in England. Dr. Brian S. Worthington, a radiologist at the University Hospital there, told me about the first images obtained in 1974.

"We were in the spectroscopy lab and had a tiny magnet. The first thing we looked at under the magnet was an onion, and we saw its inner rings. We could see water content in the tissue, too."

One of the first human MR scans in England was that of a human wrist in 1977.

"The first experimenters had great concerns about what the magnet might do to humans," Dr. Worthington recalled. "I remember someone questioning whether we might even remove centers of memory in the brain with too strong a magnet."

In 1978 the first head scan was obtained. The doctor-scientists themselves volunteered as the first subjects. In 1980 the first patient was scanned for a brain lesion. That same year MR was introduced to radiologists at the Radiological Society of North America's meeting in Chicago in a "New Horizons" lecture. MR's application and growth have ushered in a veritable "Golden Age" of diagnostic medicine that has just begun. Its full potential is yet to be explored.

Like the director of a chorus, an MR scanner conducts the ``singing'' of hydrogen atoms within the human body.

The scanner surrounds the body with powerful electromagnets. Supercooled by liquid helium, they create a magnetic field as much as 30,000 times stronger than that of the earth.

This field has a profound effect on protons, the nuclei of hydrogen atoms. Spinning like tops, the protons normally point in random directions **A.** But inside the scanner's magnetic field **B** they align themselves in the direction of the field's poles. Even in alignment, however, they wobble, or precess, at a specific rate, or frequency. The stronger the magnetic field, the greater the frequency (f+).

When the scanner excites these protons with a radio pulse timed to the same frequency as their wobbling, it knocks them out of alignment **C.** Within milliseconds they spiral back into place **D,** singing out with a faint radio signal of their own.

A computer translates these faint signals into an image of the area scanned (diagrams on facing page). The image reveals varying densities of hydrogen atoms and their interaction with surrounding tissues in a cross section of the body. Since hydrogen reflects water content, doctors can use the image to make distinctions between tissues.

Scientists picked hydrogen as the basis for MR scanning because of its abundance in the body and its prominent magnetic qualities. Research is also under way on employing other elements, such as sodium or phosphorus, whose altered properties could provide early warning signs of strokes or heart attacks. It may even become routine to tag cloned antibodies with a detectable element, giving scientists a powerful tool to study such disorders as diabetes, allergies, infertility, and cancer.

A
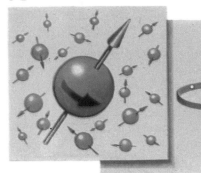

B
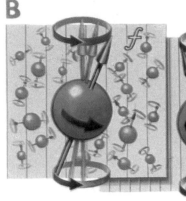

C
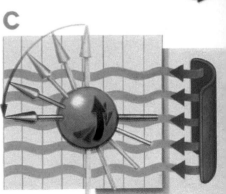

D
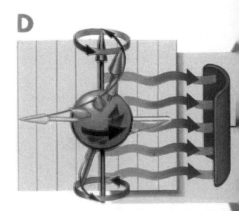

1

To make an image (oval at center of page), the computer establishes a grid of tiny boxes, or voxels, in three dimensions, X, Y, and Z. First the magnetic field is varied in the Z direction, from head to toe, to define a plane of interest (orange disk) where the body will be scanned. Within this plane protons wobble at a given frequency, f. Radiofrequency (RF) coils then emit a pulse at precisely the same frequency to topple these protons.

2

Before the protons can realign themselves, other coils briefly vary the magnetic strength of the plane in the Y direction. This causes protons to wobble at different rates (clock faces) from the top of the plane to the bottom. Detecting these differences over hundreds of pulse-and-response cycles, the computer locates voxels in the Y direction.

3

Coils then vary the magnetic field from left to right in the X direction, causing protons to sing at different frequencies as they realign themselves. Having located each voxel in the X, Y, and Z directions, the computer assigns each voxel a spot on the video screen. The spot's brightness is determined by the number of protons within the voxel and the magnetic properties of the tissue. Together the dots form a readable image.

Very few developments in medicine have proceeded as quickly as MR. Dr. William Oldendorf at the University of California in Los Angeles feels that "in our current analysis of MR signals, we are probably at the level of Marconi in 1901 when he first spanned the Atlantic by radio."

With MR scanners we are looking at the alignment of the proton in the hydrogen atom. But what about imaging other chemical elements? The brain contains phosphorous. Biologic energy is stored in molecules that contain phosphorous and is released when needed. It is the basis of the living system. If we knew the amount of energy-rich phosphorous molecules in the brain, it would help us in understanding more about the brain's functions.

We know too that the brain generates electrical energy and that a current flow exists throughout the entire nervous system. That current flow has a magnetic field (measured in Tesla, a unit of magnetic field strength. It is about 10^{-13} Tesla in the body; the earth's field is about 10^{-5} Tesla). If we can measure this energy, find out where and how it varies, it might prove useful in understanding many aspects of the brain's function. An immediate application would be in treatment planning for epilepsy where electrical energy malfunctions in certain brain centers can result in seizure.

Already we can differentiate the brain's gray matter (nerve cells) from the brain's white matter (nerve fibers). Since gray matter contains 15% more water than white matter (87% water vs. 72% water), and MR is looking at H_2O (water) protons, a great difference in contrast between the two is seen on the MR scan.

MR is useful in multiple sclerosis because the fatty tissue that normally exists around nerve fibers deteriorates and these abnormal fat-free areas can be clearly imaged.

These are but a few of the new areas of research in the field of MR imaging. Having established a firm basis for future research, physicians and scientists now look toward MR spectroscopy and the analysis of numerous chemical elements found in the human body to aid in the study, diagnosis, treatment, and cure of a host of human maladies.

A color enhanced MR image of a male patient shows tissue from the brain slumping into the base of the skull. Known to produce exquisite pictures of the brain, MR employs radiowaves and a strong magnetic field in combination.

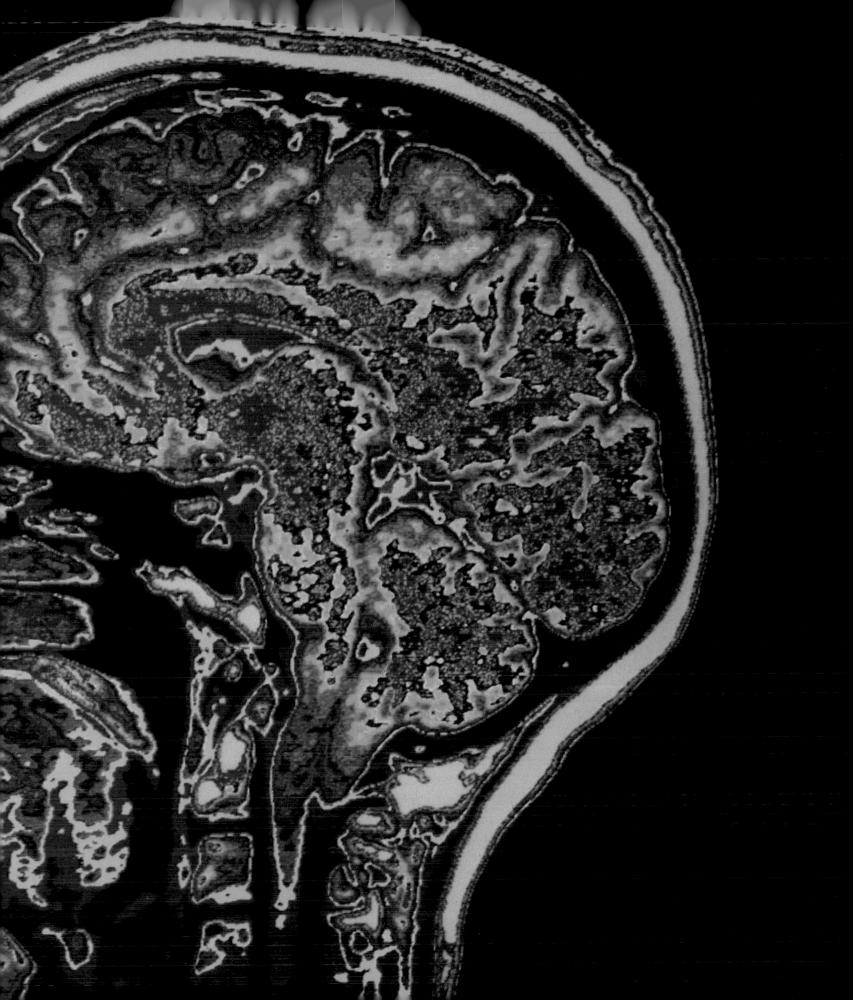

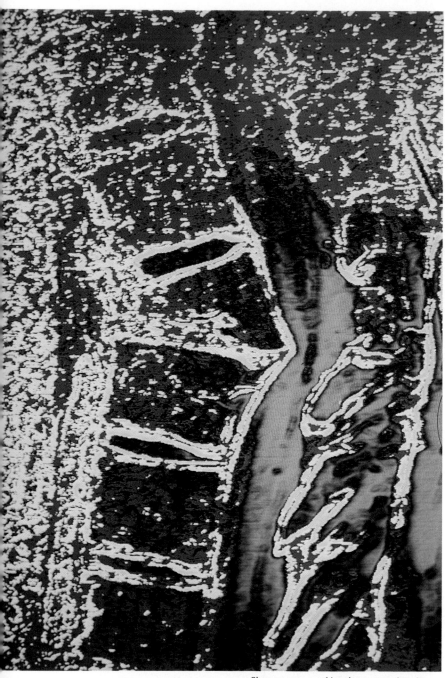

Sharp corner of broken vertebra in lower spine pushes into the nerve bundles of the spinal cord in this enhanced MR scan. Surgery could possibly restore function to the lower body of this young man injured in a motorcycle accident.

In order to tailor the approach to each patient, several facets of imaging "technique" must be considered.

First the magnet must be adjusted for the weight of each patient. The position of the patient under the magnet and/or surface coil of the radio frequency transmitter is critical. A decision must also be made as to sagittal, coronal, or axial scanning, the depth of each scan, the separation between slices, and the number of scans. There, too, the field of view of the scan, from 6 cm (2½") to 60 cm (24"), must be determined.

As a patient you may hear the radiologist mention the terms T1 and T2. When I first asked about these symbols (visible on the right side of the MR images), I was told that it was just too complex to explain. But it isn't. T1 refers to the time it takes for the atom to recover or to return to its original longitudinal alignment after the radio frequency has upset it; T2 refers to the decay of the transverse signal over a given time. Since the radio frequency signal goes on and off about every 1/25th of a second and this can be altered, a great variety of options are available to the radiologist.

Each tissue type in the body has a different T1 recovery and T2 decay time. T1 recovery time in fatty tissue is faster than in muscle tissue. Fat forms a very bright image on MR. Tumors have a long T1 recovery time and often appear darker.

By rapidly turning the radio frequency on and off, some researchers are looking into the "echo time" effect which is also valuable in looking at both anatomy and pathology.

Because of the complexity of MR and its support equipment, radiologists work side by side in the MR lab with physicists.

Working with radio frequencies can cause a host of problems, and physicists and radiologists have come up with some interesting solutions. When their first MR scanner was installed at New York Hospital, Cornell Medical Center, Patrick Cahill, Ph.D. found a greatly disturbed signal. The installation had not been fully shielded and he discovered that Vatican Radio was broadcasting at the same frequency that they were using on the scanner (about 45 megahertz). Dr. Cahill quickly

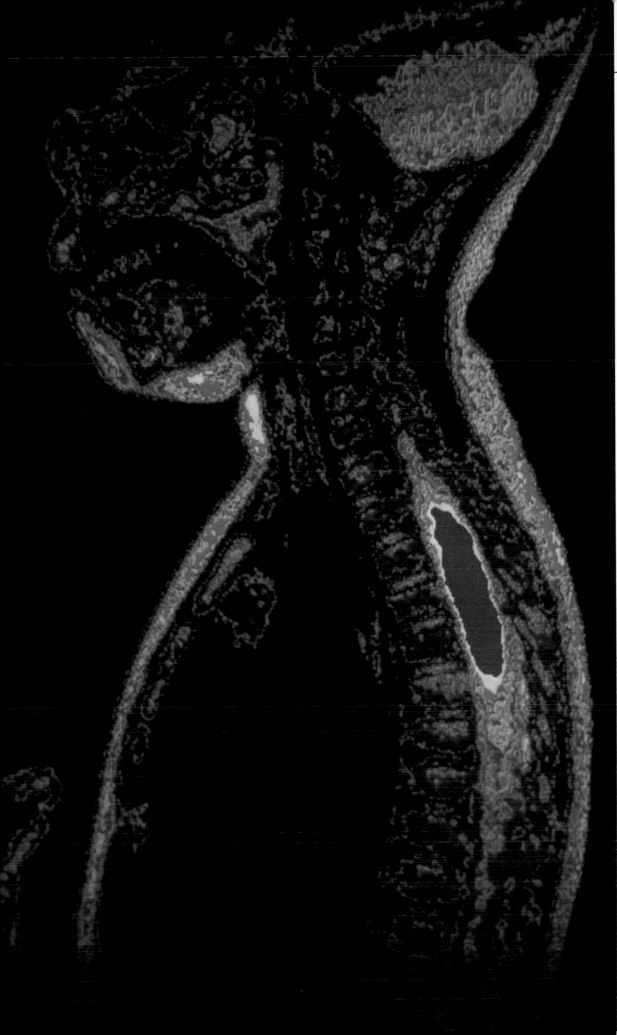

Within a week after this MR scan was obtained this 4-year-old girl lost the use of her legs. The scan showed a tumor, shaded red in this enhanced version, growing in her spinal cord. The tumor was removed and she could walk again.

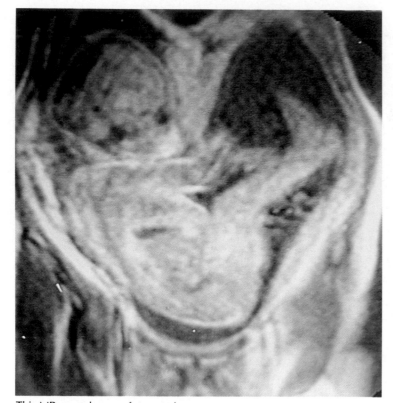

This MR scan shows a fetus at nine months, a ``breech baby'' requiring removal by cesarean section at Nottingham University, England.

shifted the radio frequency and well-defined images were obtained.

Dr. C. Leon Partain at Vanderbilt University in Nashville, Tennessee was also concerned when he found that all images produced between 2 and 3 PM were faulty. After investigating, he discovered a Ham radio operator on the Vanderbilt campus was broadcasting each day at 2 PM using the same radio frequency as the MR equipment.

Just as the technical options are varied, so too are the options available in the study of body chemistry using MR. So far the images made are studies of the proton in the hydrogen atom. Since hydrogen is a part of most organs, it is a universal imaging agent. Disease is manifested by a change in anatomy—a lesion, a tumor, or a physical change that alerts the radiologist to troubles or problems. But diseases may manifest themselves chemically long before there is an anatomical change in the body.

The body naturally ingests chemicals from air and food and digests and converts them into other chemicals for its own use. This chemical activity is an excellent indicator of body health.

It is in the study of the chemistry of the body—in metabolic and chemical changes—that MR offers great promise, and it is hoped that it will be an early detector of biochemically altered tissue. Since the early detection of diseases such as cancer may improve the cure rate, this work is important.

Dr. Nathaniel Reichek and Dr. Leon Axel at the University of Pennsylvania have been working closely in applying MR to the diagnostic evaluation of patients with heart disease. By a system of gating (synchronizing the scan with the heartbeat), they are producing three-dimensional views of the heart.

Dr. Reichek feels that in the heart MR can: 1), tell the difference between myocardium (muscle) and fat; 2), see the lumen (opening) of the arteries; 3), see reduced blood flow to the heart; and 4), measure total volume of the blood in the heart in both systolic and diastolic phases (closing and opening of heart chambers).

Dr. Axel has found that he can assess heart damage (area of infarct) since intracellular sodium gives off a different signal than extracellular sodium. Because the heart has traces of phosphorous,

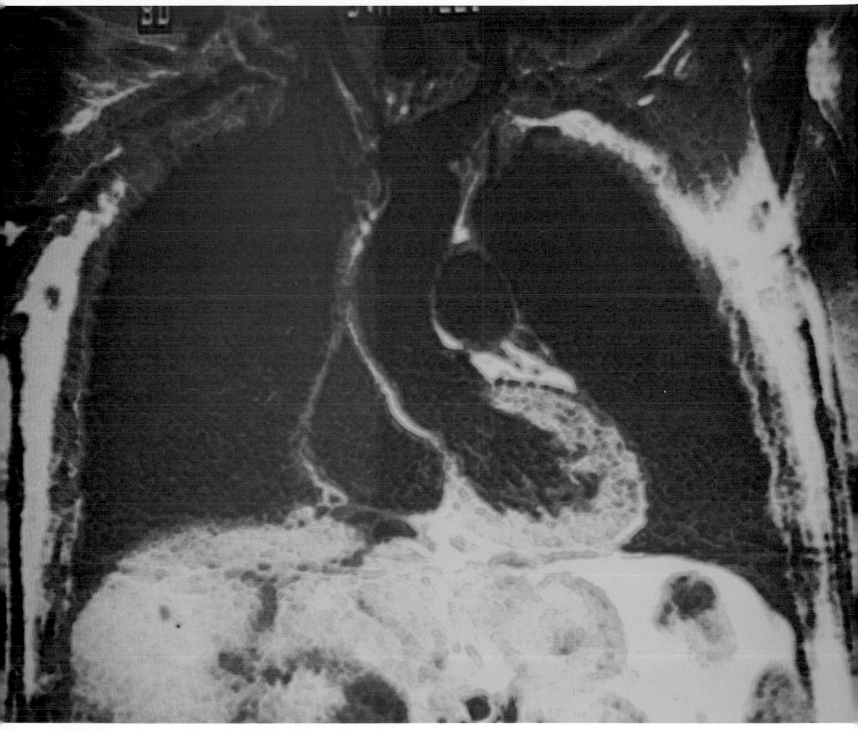

A detailed view of heart and lungs is caught in this ``gated´´
MR scan of the chest. Rib cage, lungs, and ventricles of the
heart are stopped in a single frame. Many such gated frames
put together can record the heart in motion.

sodium, fluorine, and carbon, MR will one day be used to see into the heart where each of these chemicals has a unique function.

Both Reichek and Axel are proceeding with studies on heart valve function and believe MR can be helpful in determining early rejection in the case of heart transplant patients.

"Surgery in transplants is not difficult," says Dr. Reichek, "patient management after surgery is what is difficult." Since MR is noninvasive, it is ideal in assessing postoperative progress.

"MR is like a Pandora's box. We have just opened it but don't really know where the real excitement in the field will be."

Another area of great potential for MR is in three-dimensional imaging. Since it is capable of imaging in any or all of three dimensions, it can locate and measure the anatomy very accurately. This is particularly helpful where a tumor, for instance, is wrapped around an optic nerve or is invading the spinal cord.

Some doctors now believe MR is the preferred diagnostic tool for evaluation of Alzheimer's disease and multiple sclerosis. Because there is no ionizing radiation, it is risk-free to the patient. Images can be obtained in multiple planes and MR signals from tissues are based on both chemical and physical properties which can be independently studied. Thus, in the future, it offers tremendous opportunity for early detection of disease through the study of body chemistry and function.

Along with any good comes some degree of bad, and so along with MR's wealth of benefits, naturally, comes certain disadvantages: the MR scanner works slowly (an average exam lasts 45–60 minutes, with each scan taking about 7 minutes); both the instrument and patient fee are expensive; MR cannot be used on patients with any metallic implants (i.e., aneurysm clips or pacemakers) since the images will be distorted, and the magnetic force may loosen or affect the operation of these devices; about 3% of MR patients suffer from claustrophobia and refuse to enter the scanner's tunnel.

Even so, MR is saving lives and a relatively short list of problems is a triviality to patients who have been helped.

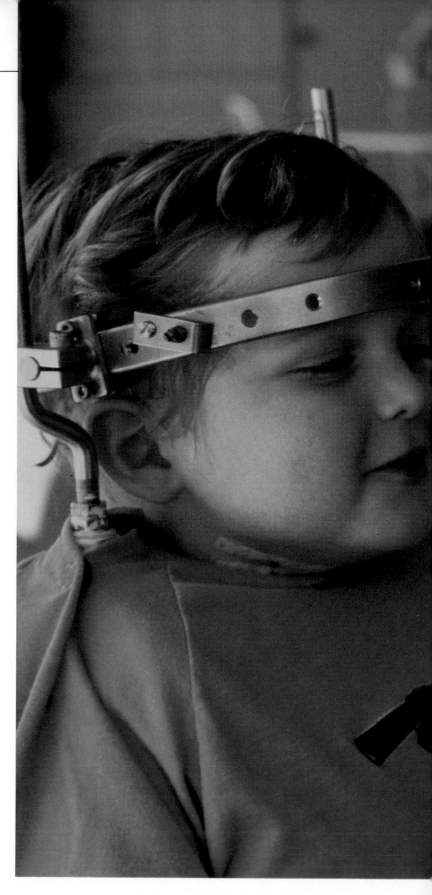

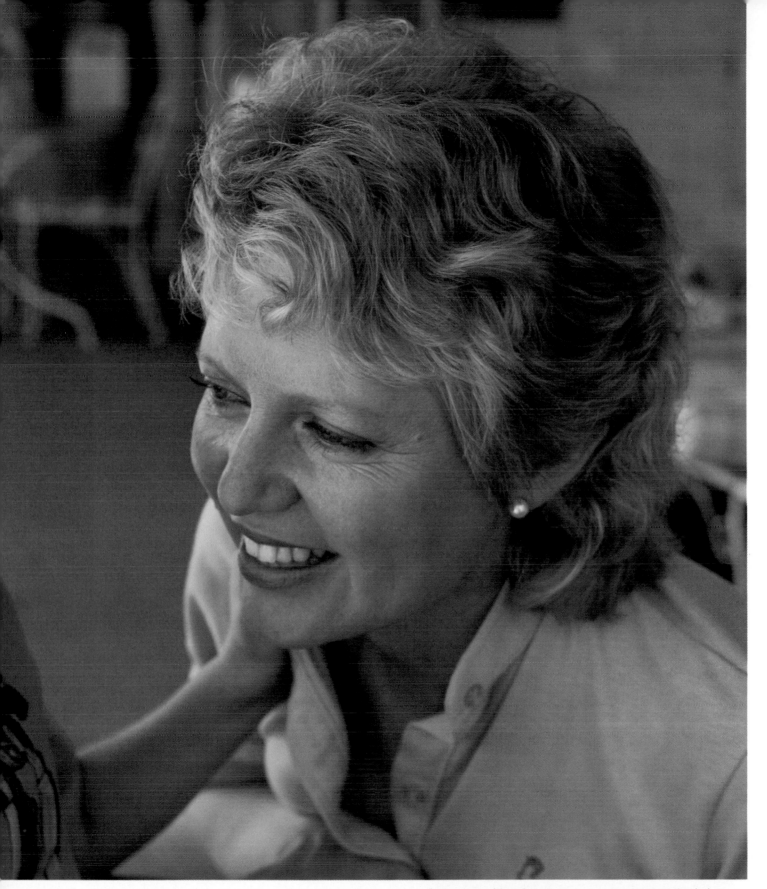

Seven-year-old Nathan Tower, wearing a supportive halo cast, is alive today because of MR scanning. When doctors in Reno, Nevada diagnosed a brain-stem tumor, ``they told us there was little hope'' said his mother, Margaret Ann (right).

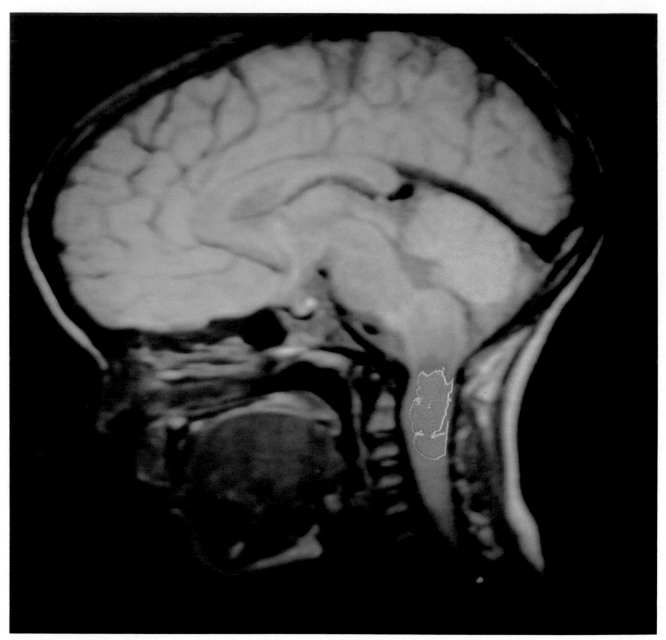

An MR scan of Nathan Tower
convinced Dr. Harold L. Rekate of
Phoenix, Arizona that the tumor
(shaded pink) could be removed.
``MR erased the bones around the
spinal cord and showed the tumor
clearly,'' said Dr. Rekate, who
performed the operation. ``Before
MR almost no one would have
attempted it.''

MR is now isolating problems never seen
before. Conditions that, in the past, were thought to
be untreatable are now being diagnosed and treated
thanks to MR imaging.

I heard about one such case and the remarkable
result from a research scientist in Milwaukee and
went to Phoenix, Arizona to get the story firsthand.

PERSISTENCE PAYS OFF

Nathan Tower is a bright, handsome boy who was born in a small town, Langley, in British Columbia, Canada. The nearest large city is Vancouver, 25 miles to the west. He is the second child of Margaret Ann and William K. Tower. Their first child, a daughter, now 13, is normal and healthy; but little Nathan experienced severe earaches as early as age two, and often threw up. As he grew older the earaches turned into headaches. His frantic mother, Margaret Ann, went from doctor to doctor trying to trace the cause of his illness. No one seemed to know. On his worst nights, Nathan was in pain from midnight to 9 AM. Aspirin provided his only relief. Nathan's health deteriorated. Over 14 doctors were consulted; the distraught mother was viewed as neurotic. Nathan lost the use of his left hand and was losing the use of his left leg. In July of 1985, Nathan was flown to Reno, Nevada for a CT scan. There was no such facility in Langley. A mass near the brain stem was discovered, but the physician called Nathan's condition hopeless because the position of the mass ruled out surgery.

Desperate, Mrs. Tower called all her geographically scattered relatives. Her husband's sister, Barbara Barnhart, lived in Phoenix. Barbara discussed the problem with a neighbor, Dr. Don Davis, who was familiar with MR imaging. He advised Barbara to have Nathan taken to Phoenix immediately and to contact Dr. Harold Rekate, a pediatric neurosurgeon at St. Joseph's Hospital.

The day after his arrival in July 1985, Nathan had an MR scan. The machine had been installed only two months earlier. "Mommy, is this a space ship?" Nathan remarked as he was positioned in the tunnel of the magnet. The images showed a clearly visible tumor lying at the base of the brain at the junction with the spinal cord. The following day in surgery, Dr. Rekate, in a delicate operation lasting more than eight hours, removed a tumor of the medulla. The tumor was 1½" long and a ½" in diameter.

Dr. Rekate explained to me that MR is unique in its ability to define tumors in the junction area between spinal cord and brain. "With MR," he said, "we are able to see brain structures we could never see before."

Several months later, I talked to Nathan and his mother on the sunny porch of Barbara Barnhart's home in Phoenix. He was wearing a "halo cast" or head brace. Additional surgery had been required to fuse the vertebrae of his neck, somewhat weakened by the first operation; the cast aided healing.

"Neurologically, he is now normal," Rekate told me later. He no longer has a weak arm or leg and, except for a stiffness in the neck, has been totally cured.

Bill Tower, overjoyed by the recovery of his son and realizing the key role that MR had played in saving his son's life, is engaged in a one-man crusade to raise public awareness and money to set up an MR center in Vancouver, British Columbia. To date, there "is not a single such installation in all of western Canada."

I first wrote about Nathan in *National Geographic* in January 1987. A year after the story appeared, I called Dr. Rekate to get an update on Nathan and the consequences of the story. Public response had been gratifying.

Dr. Rekate explained: "I did surgery on five kids who came to me because of the story. All five had tumors which had been declared inoperable: All five are now doing fine. Twenty-four others called from various parts of the country, and I referred them to competent colleagues who operated on and helped them, too. I also had a call from India, two from Norway, and another from Ethiopia."

He told me about a new technical advance, a contrast agent called gadolinium, that more clearly defines and accentuates tumors during MR scanning. He said that Dr. Burton Drayer, Chief of Radiology at St. Joseph's Hospital, is operating his MR unit 20 hours a day to keep up with the patient load and is installing a second machine. "More and more patients will be helped because of MR," he concluded.

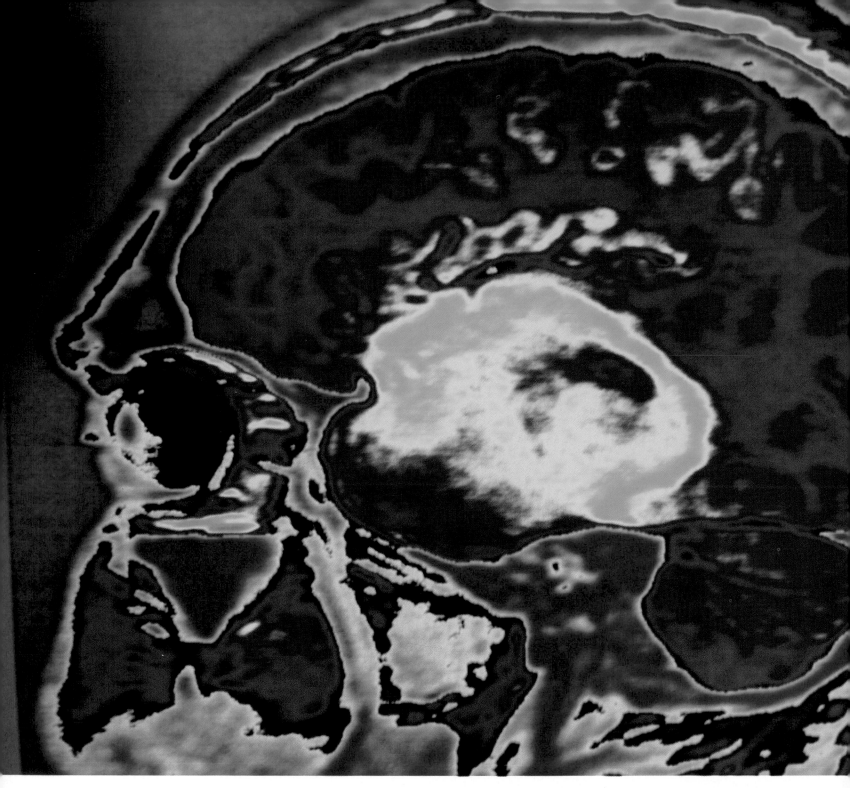

Without warning one Sunday afternoon, Joe Silvers of Tulsa, Oklahoma, fell into a convulsion at his parents' home. ``I don't even remember it happening,'' said Joe. A CT scan of Joe's brain showed what looked like a stroke. ``But that didn't make sense at all,'' said Dr. David Fell, ``especially in a healthy young man like Joe with no other neurological problems.'' An MR scan showed a tumor (tinted yellow) surrounded by fluid filled ventricles (green). Dr. Fell removed the tumor, and Joe has had no further trouble.

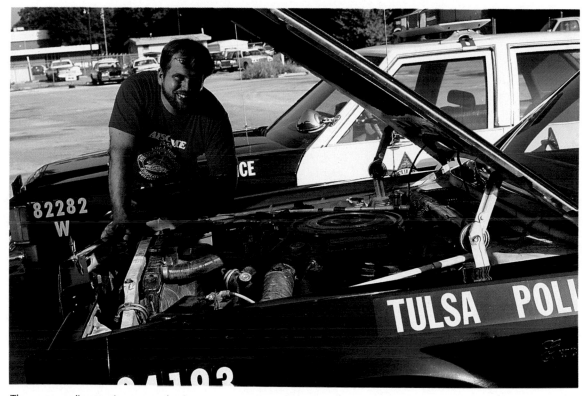

The correct diagnostic answer for Joe Silvers, who works as a maintenance mechanic for the Tulsa Police Department, came from an MR scan. Surgical removal of the tumor was followed by radiation therapy.

On a beautiful spring day, Joe Silvers and I sat on the bank of the Arkansas River just above the Keystone Dam near Tulsa, Oklahoma. We were fishing for bass and catfish. At age 33, Joe was a picture of robust good health. A slight scar above his right ear, now covered by an oversized baseball cap, was the only indication that he too had gone through a life-threatening experience.

"It was a Sunday afternoon and I had just finished a hearty meal of roast beef and potatoes, Sunday dinner with my folks," he told me. "Then all of a sudden I blacked out."

"My wife, Allison, later told me I rolled over and over on the floor and it took seven people to hold me down. It was like a fit, or being possessed, or epilepsy. I remember waking up a half hour later in an ambulance on my way to the emergency hospital. I was wide awake and felt fine."

With Joe's permission, I spoke with Dr. Clifton W. Hooser, radiologist, and Dr. David Fell, neurosurgeon, who filled me in on Joe's case.

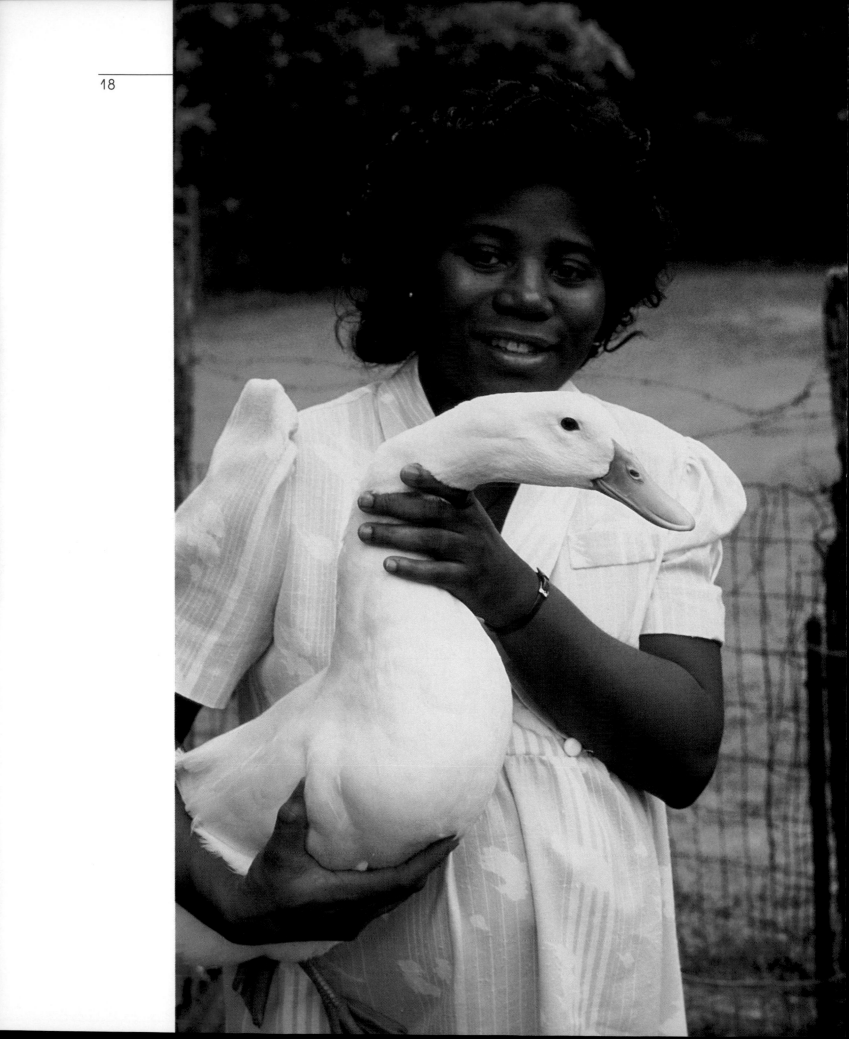

Dr. Fell began: "The attending physician ordered a CT scan of the brain, but we could see very little. We thought it might be a stroke, but at age 33 Joe should not be subject to stroke. Anticonvulsant medicine was prescribed and an MR scan was ordered for the next day."

"I performed surgery on a tumor plainly and accurately defined by the MR scan. I opened a flap about 2½" above the right ear, folded it over, and removed the tumor. It was a Grade 2 astrocytoma (brain tumor)."

Dr. Fell feels that "MR is another big leap in imaging the nervous system with precision and detail. We have had several patients with big tumors that could not have been seen in any other way, and with MR we are preventing the need for exploratory surgery and biopsy," he said.

A professor of radiology and author of several books on MR, Dr. C. Leon Partain told me about one of his patients. Wanda McClain lives in Columbia, a small town south of Nashville, Tennessee. She is married and desperately wanted a second child but could not conceive. The only symptom recorded by her gynecologist was a milk discharge from her breasts (galactorrhea). Tests showed an elevated prolactin level—a hormone that assists in the production of milk. Since it is known that pituitary tumors produce prolactin, Dr. Partain scheduled an MR scan. A small tumor was clearly visible at the base of the pituitary gland in the frontal section of the head. Dr. Cully Cobb, a surgeon at Vanderbilt University Hospital, removed the tumor by a trans-sphenoidal resection (through nose and sinus), and Wanda conceived a normal healthy child three months later.

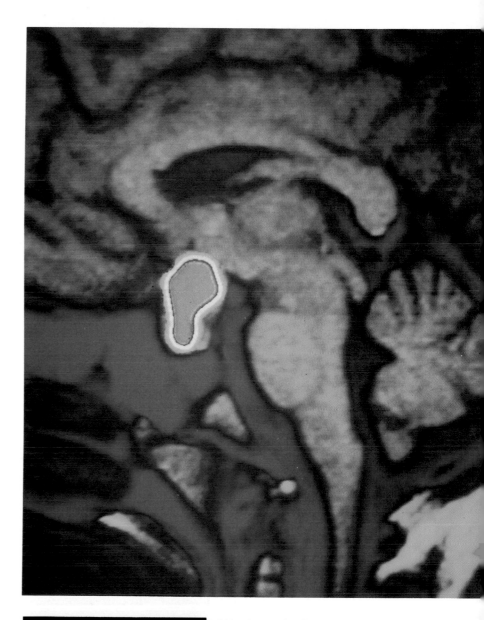

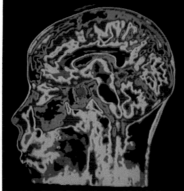

Wanda McClain lives in the small town of Columbia, Tennessee. She had one beautiful baby daughter and desperately wanted to conceive another baby. The pituitary gland when imaged by MR showed the presence of a small tumor at the base of the gland. It had caused Wanda's infertility. The tumor removed, Wanda quickly conceived a second child. Wanda, pregnant, was photographed with pet duck Jo-Jo.

I traveled to Bakersfield, California to get another story of how MR was helpful in saving the life of 4-year-old Ashleigh Slaughter. Born on June 4, 1984, Ashleigh at 5 months was in severe pain. She screamed frequently, wouldn't nurse, and could not sit upright, or sleep normally. Connie, her mother, a radiological technician and familiar with diagnostic tests, tried everything. X-rays revealed little, but an ultrasound scan indicated a tumor at the level of Ashleigh's kidney. The tumor was removed surgically, but Ashleigh still suffered. Chemotherapy was prescribed after MR finally disclosed a larger tumor that entered the spinal canal and compressed the spinal cord. Following a month of chemotherapy, another MR scan revealed a 60% shrinkage of the mass. After almost a year of intermittent sessions of chemotherapy, MR revealed no presence of the obstructing mass. Today Ashleigh is a normal, healthy, happy child.

Though embraced as a fantastic tool by radiologists, some surgeons have been slow to accept MR imaging. At the Mallinckrodt Institute in St. Louis, Dr. Klaus Sartor told me about the problems of convincing older surgeons of the effectiveness of the new technology. In a recent case, a CT scan (later confirmed by an MR scan) indicated a large brain tumor in a male patient. A famous neurosurgeon armed with these films opened the skull of the patient. While surgery was proceeding, Dr. Sartor received a call from the neurosurgeon.

"There is no indication of a tumor in the area indicated on the scan," the surgeon insisted.

Usually tumors are easily seen by the surgeon because they have a different color or texture compared with healthy, gray-white, gelatinous brain tissue. But in this case, the tumor could not be seen by the human eye.

"I have been operating for over 30 years and have never removed a tumor I couldn't see," the surgeon announced.

Dr. Sartor insisted on the accuracy of his MR scan and suggested a biopsy or evaluation of the area in question. The report confirmed the presence of a tumor, and it was immediately excised. Again, MR had given information that the experienced brain

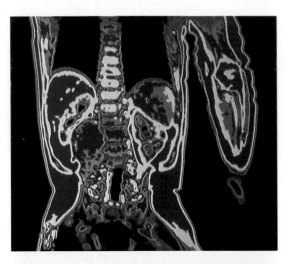

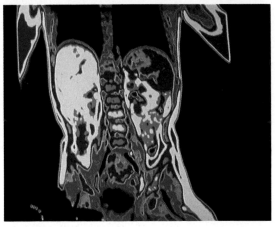

surgeon's eyes could not.

Dr. Ed Staab, Chief of Radiology at the University of Florida College of Medicine in Gainesville, confirmed Dr. Sartor's story with a similar experience.

"A surgeon feels a lesion, then operates. A surgeon sees a lesion, then operates," said Staab.

Recently in Florida a pregnant woman in her second trimester had symptoms of liver infection. An MR scan clearly revealed a lesion in the liver.

The patient's surgeon proceeded with the operation but couldn't find the lesion. "He scrubbed up twice before I could get him to believe that a tumor did exist in the patient's liver," commented Dr. Staab.

Later by phone, the surgeon confessed it was the fourth time in several months that he had seen MR images of abnormalities that were not visible at surgery.

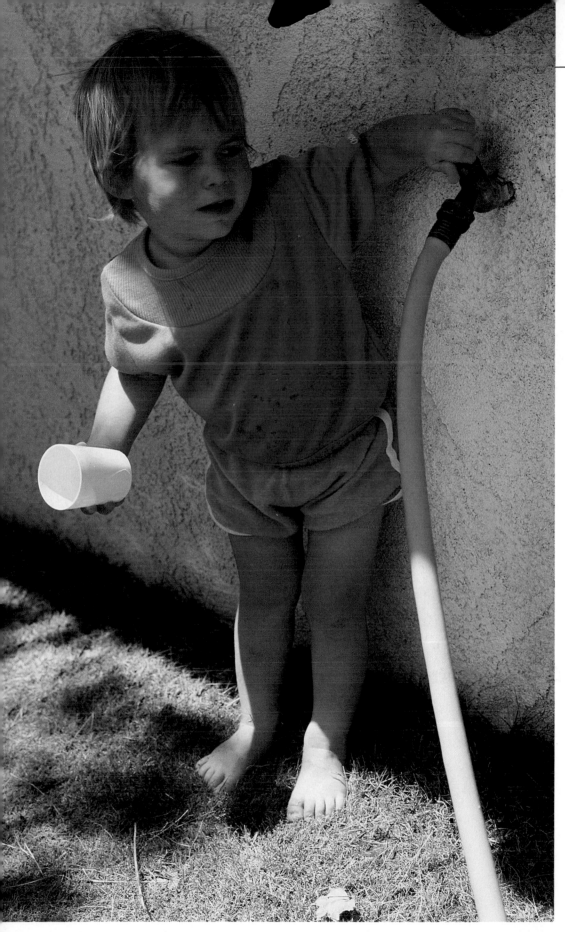

Caught in time by doctors, a malignant tumor bulges between the kidney and the spinal column of 7-month-old Ashleigh Slaughter. Appearing dark blue with green intrusions (top left) in this enhanced MR scan, the tumor is entering the spinal canal and compressing the cord. ``She was in constant pain,'' said her mother, Connie. ``She was unable to sit and slept with her back arched.''

Fearing the trauma of spinal surgery on a patient so young, doctors at UCLA used chemotherapy to shrink the tumor before trying to remove it. Ashleigh responded so well to the medicine that no surgery was necessary. The tumor vanished from her body (lower left) leaving her a healthy 2-year-old. She awaits a cold drink from the hose in her yard in Bakersfield, California.

JIMMY'S STORY

One day as I sat writing about MR, a letter came to me from a reporter on the *Phoenix Gazette*. It told how two parents had read my *Geographic* story at a time when they were desperately trying to save the life of their son James, age 12. His case was not unlike that of Nathan Tower. The letter concluded: "If you never do anything else, at least you have done a story that helped save Jimmy's life."

I went to see Jimmy and his parents, Sonia and Joseph Linares, in their modest two bedroom, frame house in Mesa, Arizona, just east of Phoenix.

At age 5 Jimmy fell off a wagon hurting his head and badly spraining his neck. About two weeks after the fall Jimmy had bad headaches, then started to throw up. His coordination of arms and legs then began to fail. In December of 1980 a CT scan hinted at a barely visible tumor at the base of the brain, and the day after Christmas, Jimmy underwent 7½ hours of surgery. A part of a tumor was removed, but CT had not accurately defined the position of the tumor, making surgery difficult.

For the next two years, Jimmy—though not perfect— was improved. The headaches cleared. A shunt had been placed in the brain for drainage, and when replacement was required in 1982, all the old problems returned. Jimmy's health deteriorated quickly. He was losing all muscle function. A second CT scan indicated that the tumor was back, and a second operation was performed in July of 1983. Mrs. Linares remembers the surgeon telling her before beginning: "He will be better off if he doesn't come out of surgery."

After surgery, Jimmy's health remained poor. He was bedridden, breathing was difficult and the headaches continued. Radiation therapy was recommended. After 6 weeks of treatment Jimmy improved, but only a little. He couldn't sleep at night, so he moved into the living room. He slept on the living room floor where he could watch taped versions of TV's *Gilligan's Island*, which he loved. For two years his mother slept with him on the living room floor, changing the tape deck and dispensing Tylenol by the gross.

By February 1986, Jimmy couldn't walk; he was losing all motor functions. "We carried him in to see the doctor," Sonia Linares told me.

"There is nothing else I can do. I cannot do surgery again. He will die in surgery," the doctor told Sonia. Finally, she asked if she could take Jimmy to another surgeon for another opinion. "Don't sell your house," he responded. "Nobody can help him. You will end up with nothing." Joseph Linares had only a modest income from his job as a manager of a grocery chain supermarket.

"We continued to live on the living room floor. We ate on the floor; we played on the floor; and, of course, there was always Gilligan," Mrs. Linares told me.

In February 1987 Jimmy choked on his dinner, and was rushed to the hospital. "Jimmy is going to die. I can only make it easier for him to die" the doctor in attendance told Sonia and Joseph. But Jimmy survived.

In April of 1987, Mrs. Linares went to visit her eldest daughter, Ginger, in Bakersfield. Ginger had read an article in the *Phoenix Gazette* telling about the *National Geographic* story and the wonders of MR.

The next day, based on information in the article, Sonia called for an appointment at the Barrow Neurological Institute at St. Joseph's Hospital and Medical Center in Phoenix.

Jimmy had an MR scan the following day and the family met with pediatric neurosurgeon Dr. Harold L. Rekate the day after that.

"I'm going to try," Rekate told them, "it's an operable tumor. I think I can help this little guy."

"For the first time in five years, he gave us hope. It was a peaceful and calm feeling," Mrs. Linares recalled.

Surgery was scheduled for May 15th, but on May 14th Jimmy went into respiratory arrest. The tumor had cut off the brain area that controlled Jimmy's breathing. Rekate decided on immediate surgery.

Mrs. Linares vividly recalls this historic day in her life: "Before the operation, Dr. Rekate came in to see me. I was in the parents' surgical waiting room with my husband and our minister. It was minutes before surgery, and the doctor's surgical team had already started preparing Jimmy. Dr. Rekate asked if we

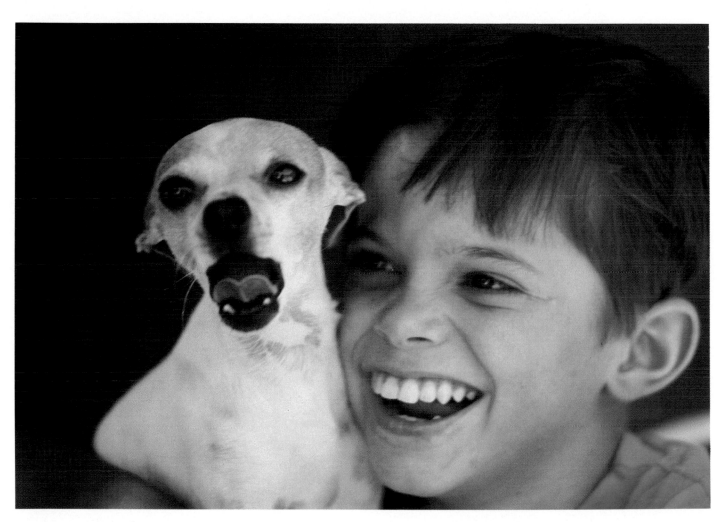

could pray. ''Please lead us in prayer,'' he asked the minister.

''The four of us held hands as the minister prayed.''

Mrs. Linares remembers telling her husband later: ''He is an angel of God. He is the man I have been praying for.'' Surgery lasted 4½ hours. Seven times during surgery Rekate had a nurse call to keep the parents posted on Jimmy's progress.

Mrs. Linares smiled. ''We gathered in Jimmy's room the next morning. Rekate jumped up after seeing Jimmy kick his right leg out (he had been totally paralyzed the day before). He exclaimed, ''Praise the Lord, this is what prayer can do. I didn't do this!''

Jimmy has had a remarkable recovery. His motor functions have been restored, and he is back at school living a happy, normal life.

Twelve-year-old Jimmy Linares in his backyard, in Mesa, Arizona, with his constant companion. After hearing about the work of Dr. Harold Rekate from a story in *National Geographic,* Sonia Linares came to the end of her search for a cure for her son.

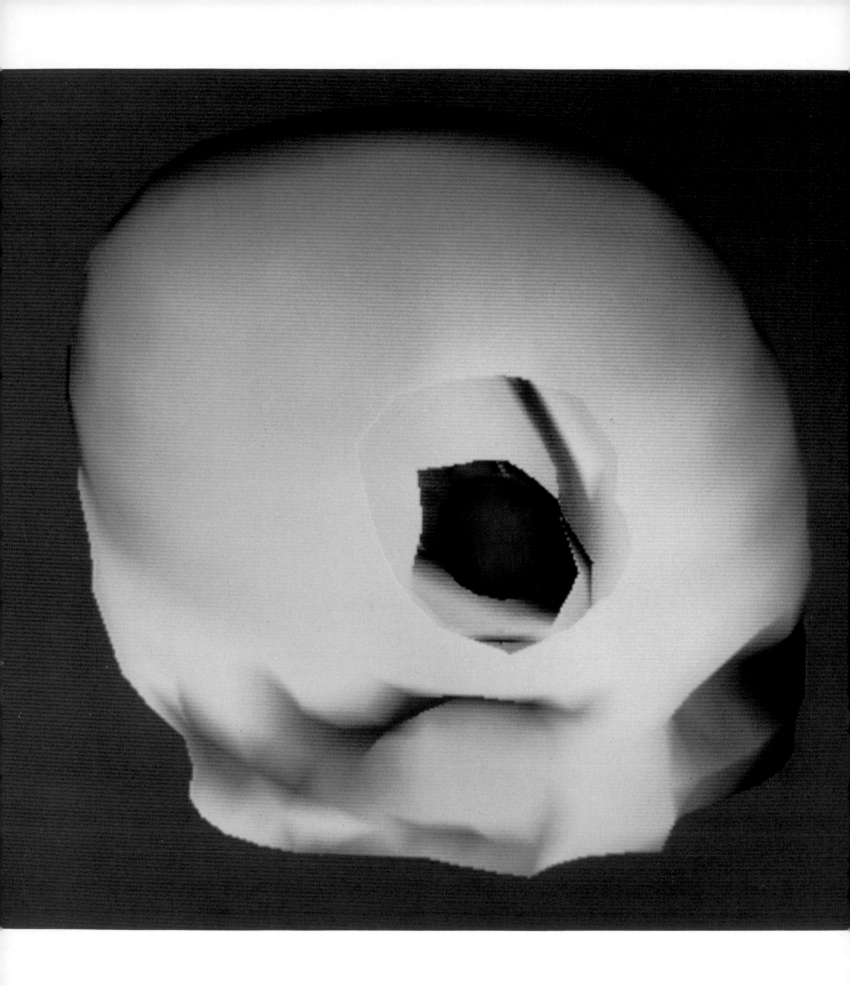

II. COMPUTED TOMOGRAPHY

"A core tool for diagnosis"

We have all had conventional x-ray studies on many occasions—for our teeth, our lungs, our broken bones— but relatively few of us have had a CT scan (also called CAT for computerized axial tomography). This imaging technique has so revolutionized diagnostic medicine in the past 15 years that there are over 5,000 scanners installed in the United States alone (about 7,000 worldwide). CT is now a core tool for virtually any diagnostic case study.

CT scanners are expensive, complex x-ray machines that use the basic principle of a two-dimensional x-ray unit but with greatly enhanced effectiveness.

X rays are produced when electrons bombard a target made of tungsten. The x rays are directed through the body where some proceed relatively unimpaired (as through body gas or air) while others are absorbed to varying degrees. Bone and muscle absorb much more of the x-ray beam than air. When the x rays are absorbed there is less exposure or shadow on the x-ray film; when the x rays pass more freely through the anatomy, as they do in passing through air, greater exposure of the film is the result. This varying degree of exposure produces a radiographic image that details the inner anatomy of the patient.

A conventional x-ray film gives the radiologist a range of about 20 to 30 gray scale variations that can be read or interpreted. These gray scale variations are directly related to the amount of film exposure.

Lurking deep within the brain, a tumor glares red in a computer-generated picture of a man who collapsed at a Las Vegas gambling table. This 3-D view, looking through the forehead, shows the skull's surface as white and the brain's surface as yellow, based on data collected by a CT scanner. Changing the face of medicine, a new generation of imaging devices enables radiologists to watch vital organs at work, identify blockages and abnormal growths, and even detect warning signs of diseases — all without exploratory surgery. This tumor was removed, and the patient recovered.

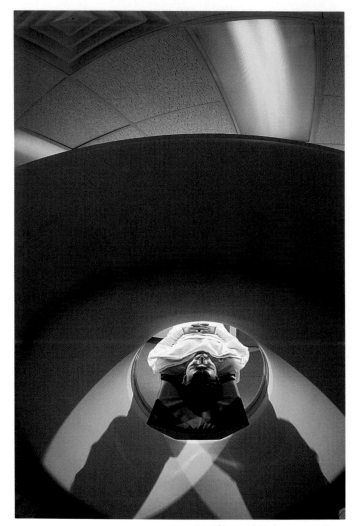

A patient lies within the donut-like ring of a CT scanner. The yoke contains an x-ray source and almost 1,000 detectors. Detail is much improved over conventional x-ray methods.

In CT the radiologist can greatly increase the gray scale variation. State-of-the-art equipment today can differentiate over 200 shades of gray.

To get first-hand knowledge of CT, I traveled to Iselin, New Jersey and talked to Dr. Wilfried Loeffler, a physicist and technical expert in CT scanning.

The equipment consists of a huge donut-like yoke with a 40" opening. The donut is about 3' thick and 5' in diameter, weighs 4,000 pounds, and costs $1,000,000. The x-ray tube is energized to 120,000 volts, spins around the yoke, and is cooled by oil, air, and water. It can produce as many as 100,000 wafer-thin images during its life span. After imaging approximately 3,000 patients, the tube is replaced at a cost of $30,000.

As the x-ray tube circles the body, a series of about 1,000 detectors (solid state crystal chips) coated with cesium iodide receive the attenuated x-ray signal that is altered as it passes through various tissues, much as a sheet of radiographic film receives the signal in a conventional system. Since the sensitivity to change in signal can be more easily detected electronically, a computer-processed image of the x-ray signal can be far superior to the conventional x-ray image. The CT scan is displayed in visual form on a monitor.

The image is usually a two-dimensional axial (cross-sectional) view varying in thickness from 1 to 10 mm. To help visualize: It would take a stack of almost 100 (1 to 2 mm) sections to form a complete crown to chin scan of the human head. The pixel (computer term for a square of information being recorded) allows the radiologist to see an area as small as 0.45 mm and a contrast difference of as little as 0.4% over the image area.

It takes the yoke one and a half seconds to spin around the patient. An average procedure with a dozen scans (or image slices) takes about 20 minutes. In a normal procedure the midline radiation dose is less than 20 mGy (an absorbed dose of radiation). This is a little higher than the dose given in your annual dental x-ray exam.

Having a CT scan is just as easy as having an MR scan as described in Chapter I. No hospitalization is required and it's done on an outpatient basis. Since

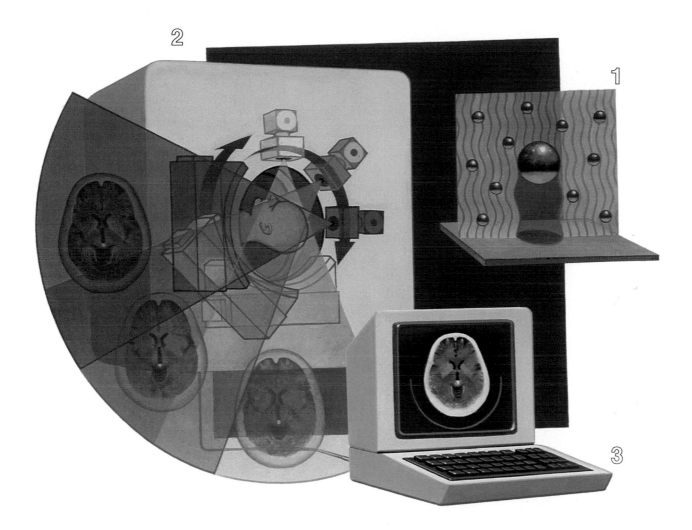

there are plenty of CT scanners in use, there is seldom a prolonged waiting time; emergency patients are handled immediately.

For a body scan, a hospital gown is worn. If the gastrointestinal tract is scanned, fasting before your appointment and evacuation of the bowel by administration of an enema are occasionally required. In 50–80% of all scans a contrast agent is administered either orally, rectally, or by injection into the vein. After the injection, some patients experience a flush or minor burning sensation, slight nausea, or a metallic-like taste.

Penetrating the body with a thin, fan-shaped x-ray beam, a CT scanner produces a cross-sectional view of tissues within. Conventional radiographs, which view the body from only one angle, can be difficult to interpret when the shadows of bones, muscles, and organs are superimposed on one another. Large molecules such as calcium absorb x rays as they pass through the body: 1) partially masking whatever lies behind them. But CT scanners allow the radiologist to view a ``slice'' of the body from many angles by moving an x-ray tube around the patient. 2) Sensitive detectors on the opposite side record what the scanner sees, and a computer 3) reconstructs the many views to make a single diagnostic image.

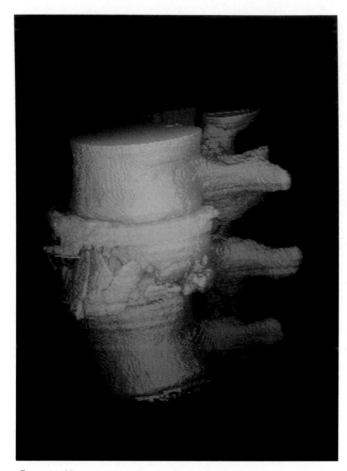

Fractured in a motorcycle accident, a young man's vertebrae seem to rise off the page in a 3-D image reconstructed from 63 CT scans. The force of the impact compressed and fragmented the vertebra at center, twisting the spine above and below it.

Developed in Great Britain in 1972, CT scanners convert x-ray pictures into digital computer code to make high-resolution video images. The computer graphics employed are similar to those used to reassemble pictures beamed back from distant space probes like Voyager. Depicting bone structures in fine detail, CT scans can also show small differences between normal and abnormal tissues in the brain, lungs, and other organs. Still in the early stages of development, 3-D CT images are beginning to play an important role in reconstructive surgery.

Optic nerve joins eye and brain

I had a CT scan done in order to better understand the procedure. After climbing aboard a table, its base was extended to place me under the yoke of the scanner. Several straps and Velcro fasteners held me in place, and I was told to remain perfectly quiet (occasionally sedatives are given to help patients relax). I had the use of a two-way intercom and communicated with the CT technician who retired to a shielded, glass-enclosed control room. No contrast material was given.

During the procedure, which lasted only five minutes, I heard humming and clicking noises as a system of gears and motors spun the x-ray tube and its matching sensor detector ring around my body. I felt no sensation and had less discomfort than experienced during a dental x-ray session where the placement of the dental films can often be uncomfortable.

The black and white cross-sectional view of my brain took less than five seconds to appear on the screen. Cut to a 1 mm slice at eye level, I could easily define the orbits of my eyes, the cord-like optic nerve, the bones of my head, and the ventricles (fluid-filled cavities) of my brain. This was a view that conventional x-ray techniques could never have produced.

The anatomy in all dimensions

A new application of CT is three-dimensional (3-D) reconstruction imaging. While CT, as described, has much improved imaging of small bones and some soft tissues, the images are two-dimensional. Radiologists are expert in interpreting CT scans and are trained to view these two-dimensional scans and conceptualize three-dimensionally, but many times the users of this information, e.g., surgeons, find interpretation difficult.

Fifty-eight CT slices were computer-assembled to produce this inside view of a man's brain. A long, tubular tumor in the vicinity of the optic nerve extends from the front of the head (right) to almost the mid-brain.

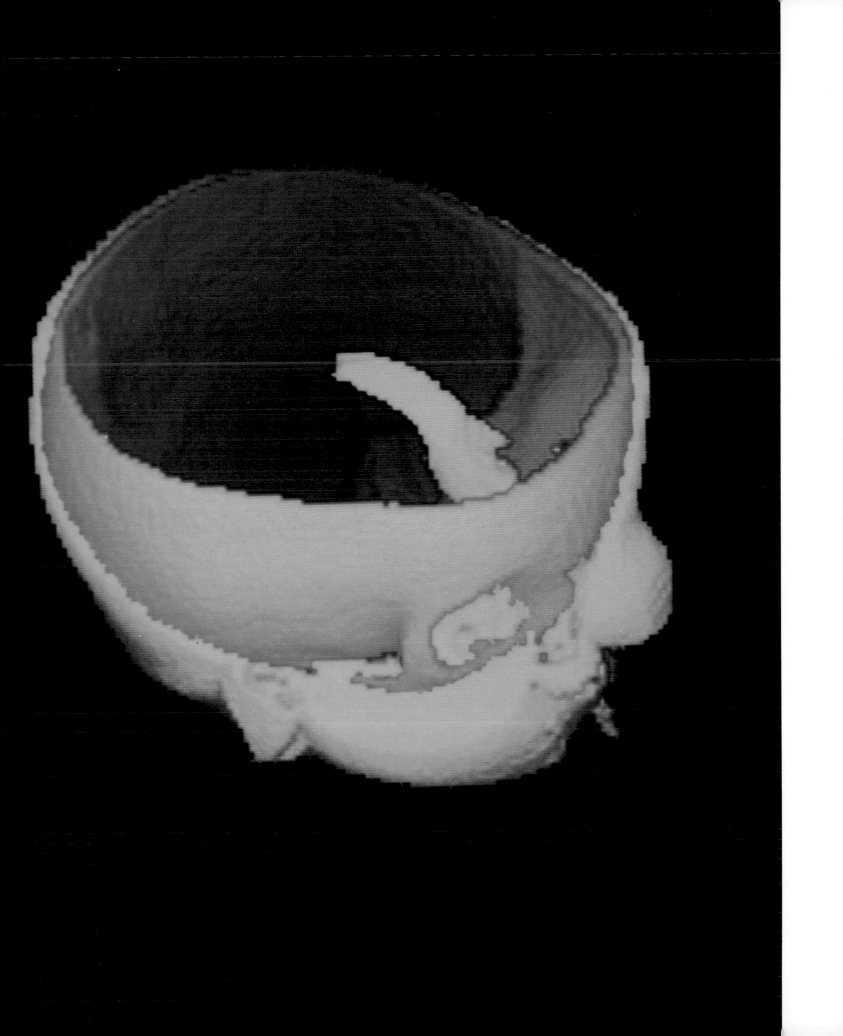

With 3-D imaging, the anatomical structure in question is viewed on a computer screen as an easily distinguished 3-D object—for example, a hip bone or skull that can be rotated in space for easy viewing from any angle or at any magnification. This development is particularly applicable in the field of cranial and reconstructive surgery, and I traveled to the Mallinckrodt Institute of Radiology in St. Louis to discuss the technique with two pioneering experts, Dr. Michael W. Vannier, a radiologist, and Dr. Jeffrey C. Marsh, a plastic surgeon.

As Vannier told the story, one afternoon he found Dr. Marsh using x-ray films of a child's head to make cutouts; the cutouts helped him visualize in three dimensions the materials he needed for bone replacement in the fractured skull.

Vannier, trained in computer design, saw the possibility of creating an exact 3-D model of the damaged skull so that Dr. Marsh could completely plan his surgery (typically, a surgeon performs multiple operations: one to assess the problem and measure the damage, a second to harvest bone from another part of the body, and a third to match and install the new parts).

Vannier went to work on his computers and devised a method of taking a number of CT images, stacking them in the computer one on top of another, and redisplaying them as a 3-D image. The results were so impressive that 3-D imaging for reconstructive surgery is now being used at major centers from coast to coast.

Rebuilding a hip joint

Another user of this technology is Dr. Steven Woolson, an orthopedic surgeon. On a sunny January afternoon he introduced me to his patient My Tien Tran, a young Vietnamese girl who was on one of the last planes out of Saigon Airport on the day before it fell to Ho Chi Minh and the communists. All her life My Tien had suffered severe pain from a congenital dislocation of her right hip. She limped and was forced to walk on crutches; her right leg was 3″ shorter than the left. Her physical disability was accompanied by much personal

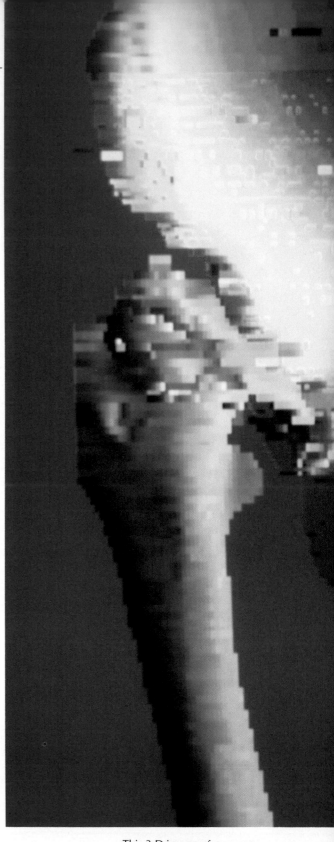

This 3-D image of a young woman's pelvis indicates a severe malformation in the right hip and a congenital (born with it) dislocation. Based on CT scans, the image was used to fashion a plastic model of the hip.

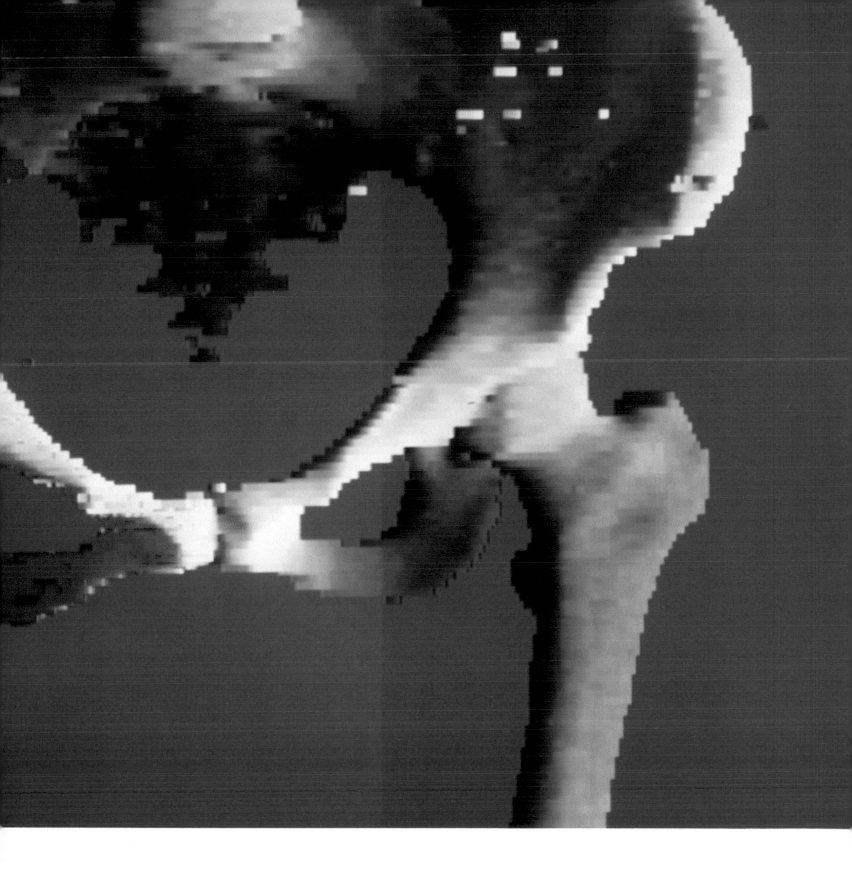

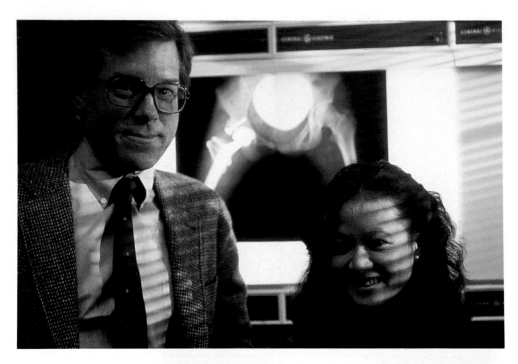

Dr. Steven Woolson and his patient, My Tien Tran, before an x-ray showing her new right hip. A 3-D image was prepared prior to surgery by Dr. Woolson. ``I wanted to be certain that the implant would fit precisely,'' Dr. Woolson said.

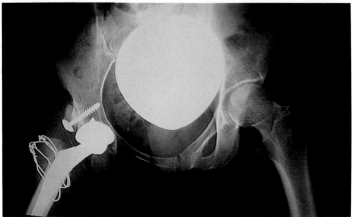

Conventional pelvic x-ray.

trauma. She married a soldier who was a wife beater; he fathered her child, and then abandoned her in Saigon.

My Tien and her daughter, Jessica, did eventually escape and some years later she came to see Dr. Woolson.

Woolson decided to do a total hip replacement. My Tien became a familiar face at the Palo Alto Medical Clinic in California, and one of the first patients to benefit from 3-D CT.

First, a series of CT scans of the hip and pelvis were obtained and used to create 3-D models of the hip bones on a computer screen. A milling machine coupled to the computer then fashioned plastic models of the replacement parts. Using these models, the surgeons determined the type and size of replacement parts (plastic or metal) that were needed. Surgery was performed and—six months postoperatively—My Tien had no hip pain, had legs of equal length, and walked normally without cane or crutches. She is now happily remarried.

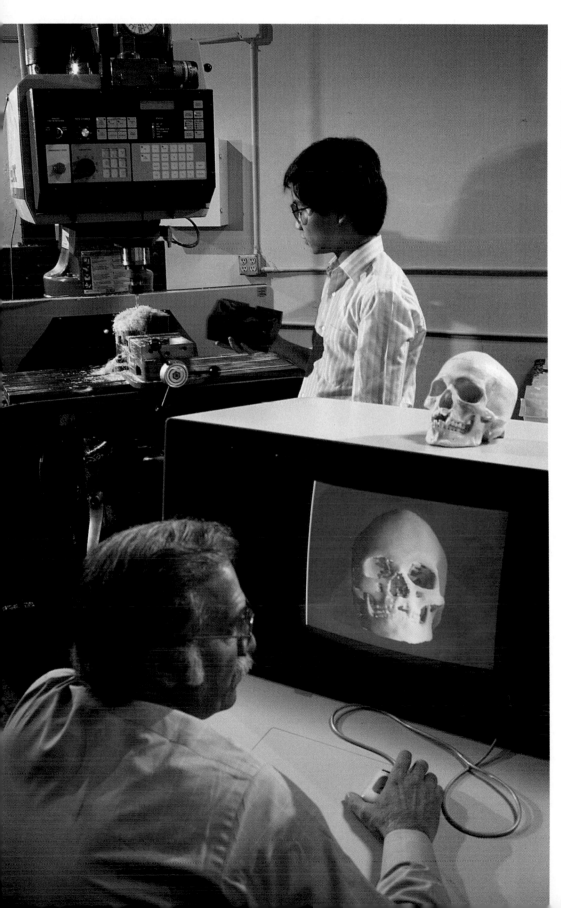

Seated at a computer console, Dr. Art Vassiliadis calls up an image from another case. The plastic skull lying on the console, like the model of My Tien's hip, was cast from a mold made on the machine in the background. Holding a block of milling wax, engineer Charles Lau helps set up the machine; its every move is controlled by the computer.

A major center for research in 3-D CT imaging is the Department of Diagnostic Radiology, University of Kansas Medical Center, Kansas City, where Dr. Larry T. Cook and Dr. Sam Dwyer have developed computer software and complex algorithms to display 3-D color images which are unique in modern medicine.

One recent assignment for Dr. Cook was to assist Dr. P. G. S. Giri from the University of Kansas, Department of Radiation Oncology. He had a patient with a tumor that was wrapped around the optic nerve of the right eye resulting in loss of vision. It is extremely difficult to perform surgery in the area of the optic nerve; one false move, a small tremor of the surgeon's knife, could cause total blindness.

Working with 30 CT scans, Dr. Cook prepared an exact 3-D model of the eye, the optic nerve, and the tumor. With the help of the model, Dr. Giri prepared a treatment plan. Result: Vision was restored, the eye saved, and the tumor greatly reduced in size. In this case, 30 scans, computer clustered in 3-D, had provided a guide for radiation therapy.

A tumor (in red) is precisely located in relation to the eyes and optic nerves in this image prepared using 52 CT scans; the rays represent possible approach routes for radiation therapy.

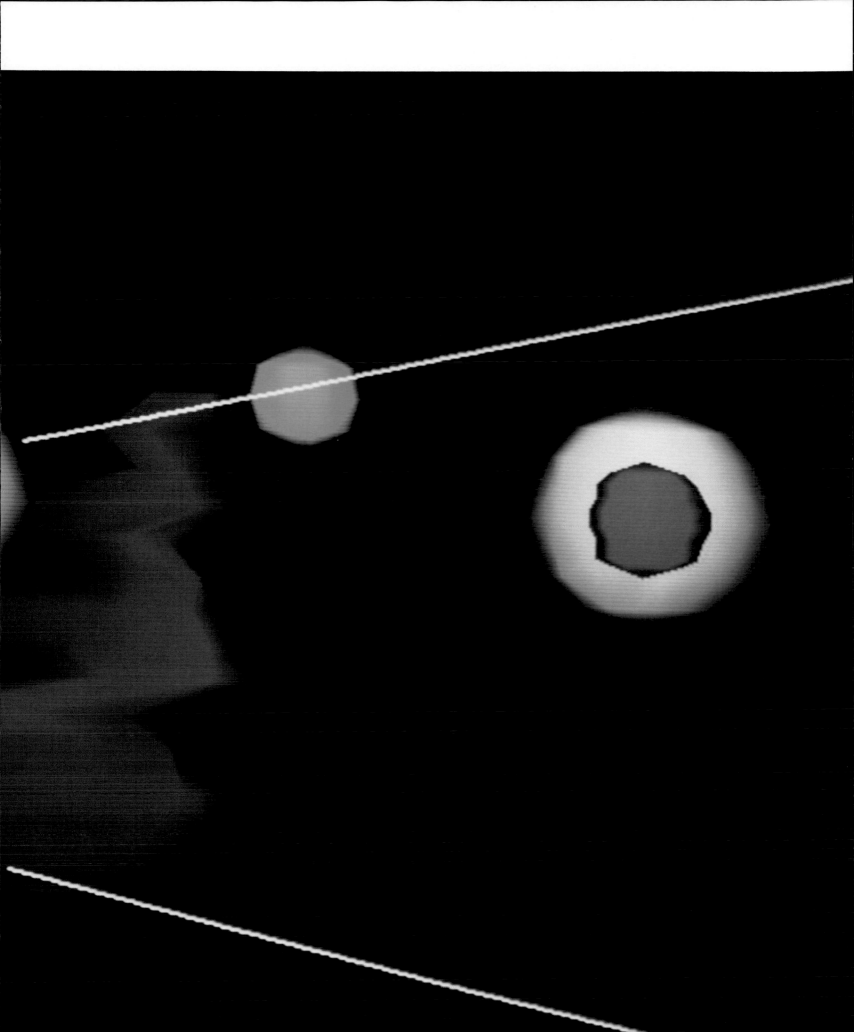

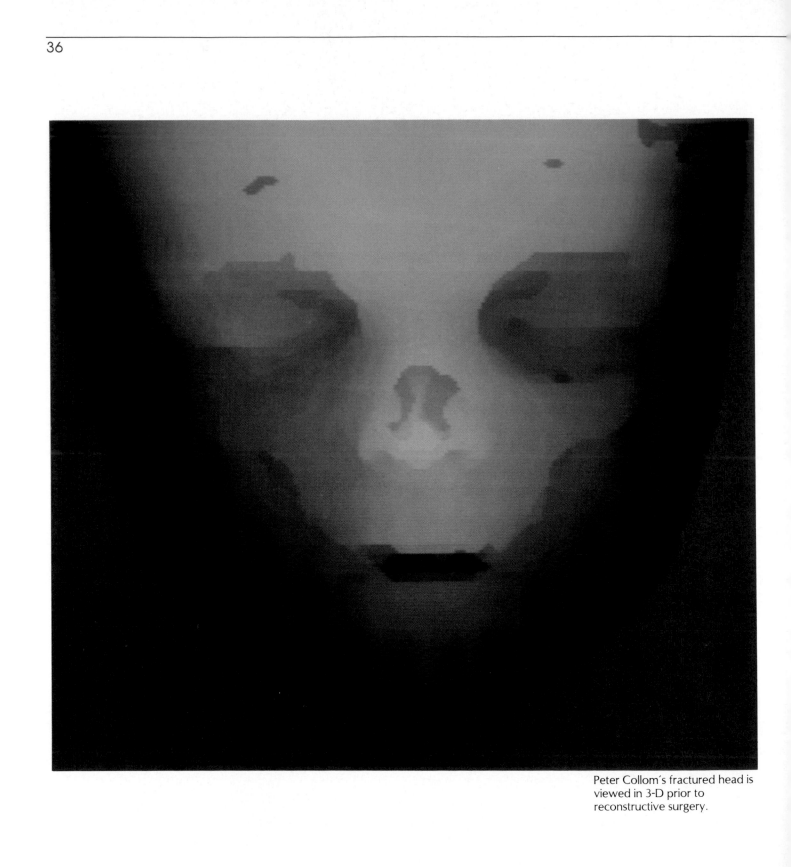

Peter Collom's fractured head is
viewed in 3-D prior to
reconstructive surgery.

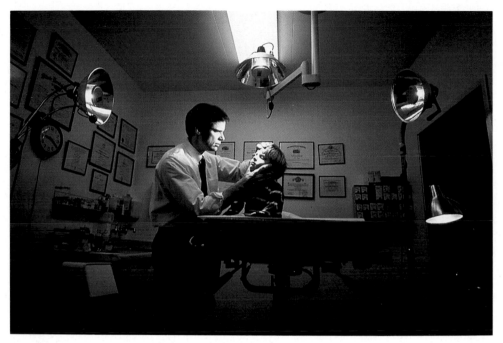

Dr. David White of Palo Alto, California operated on Peter Collom to repair his injured skull. Here he examines Peter several weeks after surgery.

Reconstructing a crushed skull

Another patient who greatly benefitted from the precise images provided by 3-D CT is five-year-old Peter Collom of Redwood City, California.

A normal, red-blooded, rambunctious boy, Peter went exploring during a visit to the library. He crawled high on a shelf and fell while reaching for a book—the bookcase and its contents tumbling after him—crushing his skull.

Dr. David White, a young reconstructive surgeon at the Palo Alto Medical Clinic, treated Pete as best he could in the Emergency Room. He later used an exact 3-D model of the child's head taken from a series of CT scans to plan his surgery. Today, Pete is fine and shows no signs of head abnormality or deformity of any kind.

From Hollywood to hospital

In a strange twist of events, equipment once used to create the mind-boggling effects for movies such as George Lucas' *Star Wars* is now being used to save human lives. The Lucas computer was especially designed to process graphic images; a modified version is now being sold to hospitals that require a quickly processed 3-D image from their CT scans.

CT now accomplishes myriad tasks that were difficult, if not impossible, on traditional x-ray equipment. It images bones exceptionally well. Because of its high resolution, minute fractures of the spine or other bones are now more easily detected. Also, gray matter in the brain can be differentiated from white matter, and white matter from cerebrospinal fluid. Hemorrhage is easily differentiated from edema (swelling), and the pancreas—hitherto almost impossible to image—is easily defined. CT helps the radiologist see foreign bodies in soft tissue, enlargement of pulmonary arteries, and hard tissue lesions. With the use of iodinated contrast material, CT can be used to evaluate blood vessel occlusions. It is useful postoperatively in imaging vein grafts and assessing the success of coronary bypass surgery.

The "C" in CT, as we know, stands for computer or computed. It is the computer that makes the whole process possible; it is the "heart"

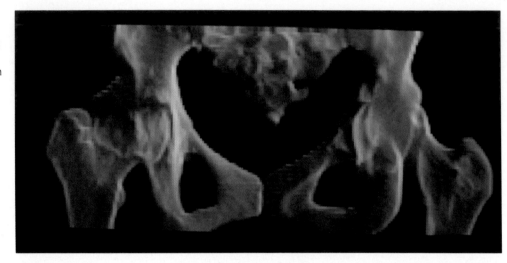

A computer developed for Hollywood movies is ideally suited to medical imaging. This 3-D view was prepared by Dr. Elliot Fishman at Johns Hopkins Hospital in Baltimore.

of modern radiology and the imaging process. What was first devised and used in England in 1969 by Geoffrey Hounsfield, a physicist, and John Ambrose, a neuroradiologist, has revolutionized medical diagnosis and the profession of radiology.

In a CT scanner the computer is the interface with the human operator: it controls the scanner, acquires the data, processes, displays, and stores the image, and archives the data. By typing on the computer's keyboard the operator enters necessary instructions to the machine: slices required, thickness of slices, voltages and current amounts. The patient's personal information is also recorded.

Several million bytes (units) of information are assessed per second as the yolk spins around the patient. The x-ray source is pulsed as it moves to keep radiation exposure at a minimum, while the output of each of the thousand electronic detectors is read independently. The data are then edited and corrected by the computer and an image is displayed. The radiologist can alter brightness and contrast, and zoom into specific areas—magnifying as well as reducing image size.

Once the image is processed it can be stored in several ways. A permanent film (or hard copy) of the image can be made, or the image can be stored in the computer memory disc or on magnetic tape. The latter has become a preferred method, since many medical professionals might simultaneously need to access the same images at various hospital locations.

One of the most active centers for state-of-the-art CT technology is the Radiology Department of Johns Hopkins University in Baltimore, Maryland. There, Drs. Elliot Fishman and Donna Magid have pioneered new uses and applications for CT imaging on a routine basis. Working mainly on orthopedic cases, they have developed algorithms and computer software, and obtained thousands of 3-D studies of hips, shoulders, knees, and spines of over 800 patients. Using as many as 85 slices (4 mm in thickness and overlapped every 3 mm, or even 1.5 mm thick and overlapped every 1 mm), they can display a 3-D image in less than two minutes.

Dr. Fishman has also experimented with ionic and nonionic contrast agents that enhance contrast in soft tissues that are presently difficult to image. Nonionic contrast material has proved to cause fewer patient reactions or side effects.

One hundred patients a day are imaged on the four Hopkins' machines; about 55% are outpatients, and 45% are hospital patients. Dr. Fishman uses dual-energy equipment that—when set at different voltages (usually 85 or 125 kVp)—can even detect the composition of such things as kidney stones. This is very important in treatment. For example, lithotripsy (see Chapter V) is ineffective with oxalate stones (salt of oxalic acid) but is effective with stones formed from uric acid salts.

Three-dimensional CT imaging is used at Johns Hopkins by one of its brilliant reconstructive cranial surgeons, Dr. Craig DuFresne. A recent case involved Siamese twins from Germany who were joined at the head. There are quite a few Siamese twin cases in the world, but most cannot be separated without sacrificing one twin.

In this case, Dr. DuFresne traveled to Germany with several colleagues from Johns Hopkins and found, by studying the CT and MR scans, that two separate and distinct brains existed. The circulatory systems of the twins, however, had to be separated and reconstructed.

He returned to the U.S. with a series of CT scans. Three-dimensional images were made and the exact skeletal replacement parts needed were milled from titanium, which is used because it has an electromagnetic field capability of its own that attracts and enhances bone formation. The 3-D models prevented the need for exploratory surgery and the standard carve, chip, and sculpt method of bone replacement.

Subsequently, the twins came to the United States for their first operation. Dr. DuFresne stood by with his models, replacement parts, templates, and even two doll models taped together at the head with Velcro.

Unfortunately, the trauma of surgery caused extensive swelling of both brains and the skulls could not be capsuled. In a second operation six months later, the plates were exactly fitted into the skulls of each child.

Dr. DuFresne now uses 3-D images routinely in his work. He offers hope to patients who come to him from all over the world and looks to the time when 3-D CT with its remarkable ability to image bone structures will be integrated with MR and its ability to produce superior images of soft tissues — also in 3-D. These techniques combined with cerebral angiography (which produces useful images of blood supply within the brain) will foster the surgeon's ability to analyze and preplan his surgical approach. All this would, of course, be cost effective since any saving in surgical time results in huge savings to the patient.

Dr. DuFresne finished his interview with me by saying: "With these new tools I can offer people

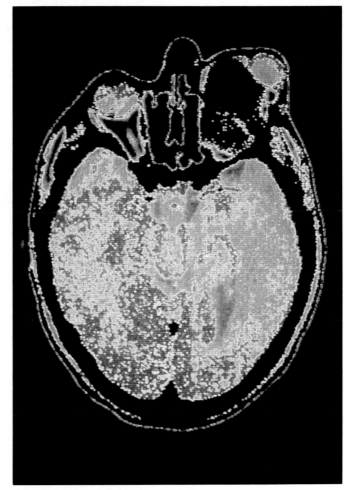

A tumor pushes out the eye socket in this image-enhanced, 2-D view of the eyes and brain in cross section.

A 3-D CT-enhanced sagittal (side) view of a man with a brain tumor (shown in red). A plum-sized tumor lies below the blue and green ventricles of the brain. Now 90 years after the discovery of the x ray, CT technology gives a more precise view of human anatomy.

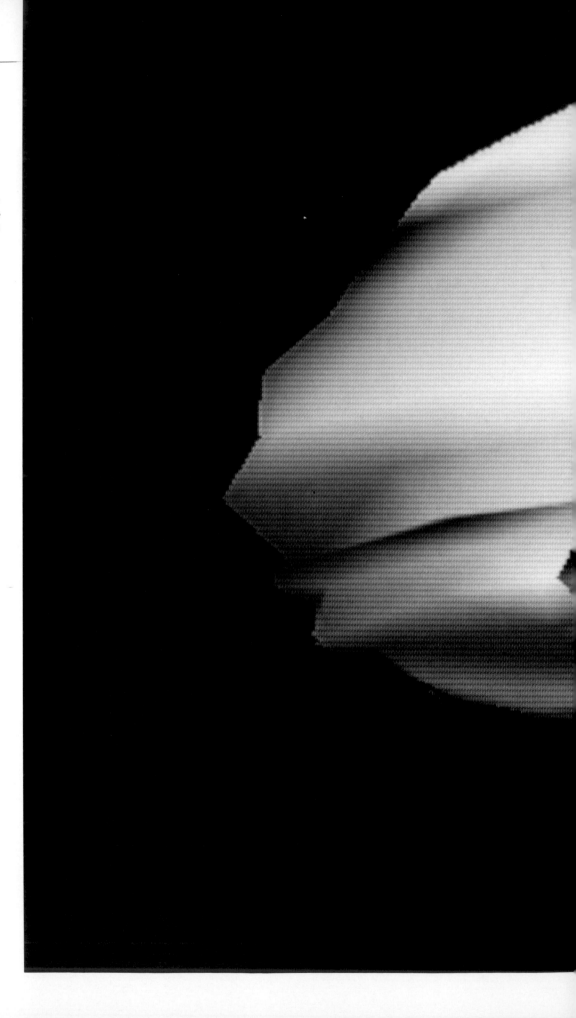

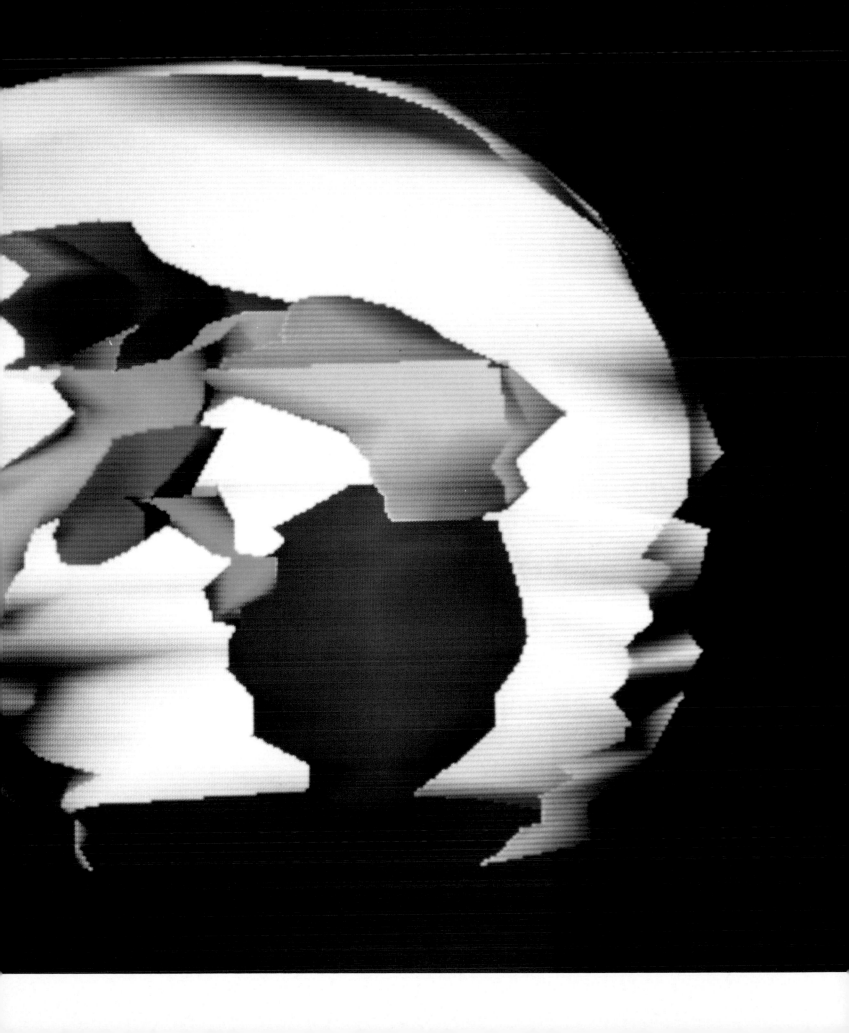

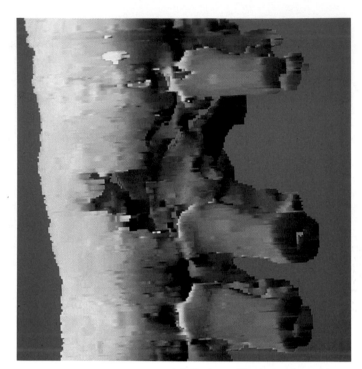

A 3-D view of human spine with fractured vertebrae. The spine was rebuilt with bone from the hip of the same patient.

with conditions that were declared inoperable some hope. I can also use these images in communicating with my patients so that they, for the first time, can easily see the problem and how I intend to proceed. Three-dimensional images are invaluable, too, in teaching the procedures to students and other surgeons."

Dr. Alec J. Megibow, an Associate Professor of Radiology at NYU Medical Center in New York, has used CT for 15 years, still remains excited and fascinated by its potential and feels it is the real work horse in diagnosis. His area of expertise is CT of the stomach, intestines, liver, pancreas and kidneys (body CT).

Dr. Megibow has lived through four generations of CT scanners: The first (in 1974) had a tube that moved in a straight line across the body, made a turn and moved back again in a straight line parallel to the first, and took five minutes to complete a scan; the second generation involved a collimated fan beam that cut the scan time to 20 seconds; the third generation had a spinning tube and fixed detectors; in fourth generation CT, both the tube and detectors spin, and acquisition time is now a fraction of a second.

Today, Dr. Megibow's department does about 500 scans weekly in both inpatient and outpatient facilities. Each of his four machines has three assigned personnel: a nurse who attends the patient, a technician who sets up the scanner, and a second technician who handles hard copy printing, film processing, and record keeping.

"Every step of the procedure is terribly important to the result," Dr. Megibow insists. "Most people see radiology as a 'black box' procedure; you press some buttons and out comes an image. Of course it's not. It takes extreme care in positioning the patient, programming the equipment, x-ray voltage, slice thickness, administering the proper kind and amount of contrast material, properly processing the images, and then carefully interpreting the finished image. I've logged a lot of miles on my eyes, but I still get blown away every day by these images. There is often such an exquisite demonstration of a disease. I ain't been bored yet."

Megibow added to my previous list of what body CT is best at: pancreatic disease, jaundice, bile duct obstruction, and problems in the abdomen, bowels, and lymph nodes.

Working with his colleagues at University Hospital in the last few years, he has discovered over 40 cases of renal cancer (malignant kidney tumors), the greatest percentage of which were discovered while performing CT for other reasons. "In these cases we found life-threatening cancer where there were no other symptoms," Dr. Megibow told me.

One of the most recent cases where CT helped save a life was in a 65-year-old woman admitted to the hospital in severe pain. The diagnosis was pancreatitis—an inflammation of the pancreas. She was sent to Dr. Megibow for a CT scan. As we talked, he displayed the films in question. In the center of one film a thin line arched around the perimeter of the pancreas near the aorta, the large vessel that distributes arterial blood to every part of the body. To me it meant little, but to him it was extremely significant.

Explaining the case, Megibow told me that the pancreas produces an enzyme (pancreatic juice) that passes into the duodenum where it plays an important role in digestion. If the pancreas ruptures (as it had in this case), the enzyme leaks into the abdominal cavity and digests anything it can find. Here it had started digesting the wall of a major blood vessel, creating an aneurysm and causing blood to spill into the abdominal cavity. The pencil-thin line was a sure sign of rupture and leakage to Dr. Megibow. "It's like putting a knife through the aorta when this happens. The patient, if not treated, would have died in a matter of four to five hours."

Thanks to a quick diagnosis, the patient was rushed to surgery and today she is recovered and doing fine.

Dr. Megibow summed it all up beautifully: "As we become more knowledgeable in reading images, and every day we do, you will find that CT is going to be the work horse in the department. It is fast becoming the evaluation method of choice. Already I hear the phrase, 'Why do a traditional x-ray?' As we progress, we are getting more bang for the buck."

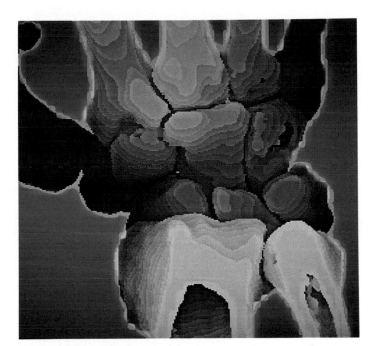

Detail of the bone structure of the right wrist. The computer assembled many x-ray images into one 3-D picture. This procedure is useful in cases of bone deterioration, inflammation, or fractures.

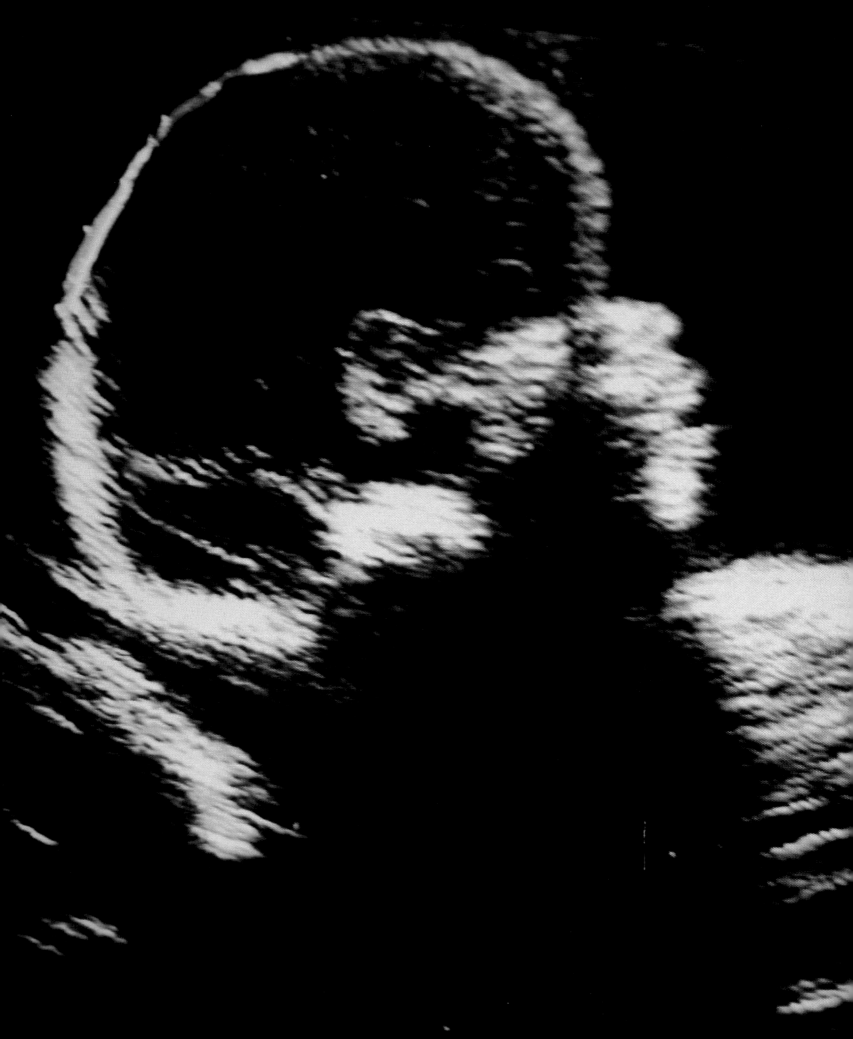

III. ULTRASOUND

"Seeing with sound"

y earliest remembrance of a doctor is a grandfatherly man in a white coat with a stethoscope dangling from his neck. I remember him gingerly thumping my chest with his fingers while listening carefully. This technique is called percussion, where air or fluid-filled spaces in the body can be detected by a difference in sound when the skin surface is tapped. It has been used by doctors since at least the eighteenth century.

The most modern use of sound in medical diagnosis is sonography or ultrasound (US) imaging, and the images it produces are unique: I saw and heard my own blood flowing through the carotid artery in my neck; watched a human fetus suck its tiny thumb, withdraw it, and give a wide-mouthed, stretching yawn; and watched as a famous neurosurgeon located a brain tumor with a baton-like probe that slowly followed the contours of a shimmering, open brain.

US is one of the simplest and least expensive imaging techniques available to the radiologist today. In clinical use for about 20 years (some of the first US images were produced at the National Institute of

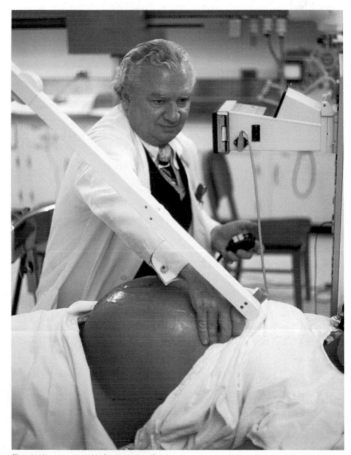

Considered safer than x-rays for use on pregnant women, sonography works like sonar to create pictures such as this view of the head of a healthy 18-week-old fetus. Usually viewed in black and white by a radiologist, this image, like most in this book, has been color-enhanced.

Dr. Lajos von Micsky, an early pioneer (now deceased), using ultrasound at St. Luke's Hospital in New York to check fetal position. He fostered the development of a sonoendoscope which reaches inside the body for internal scanning.

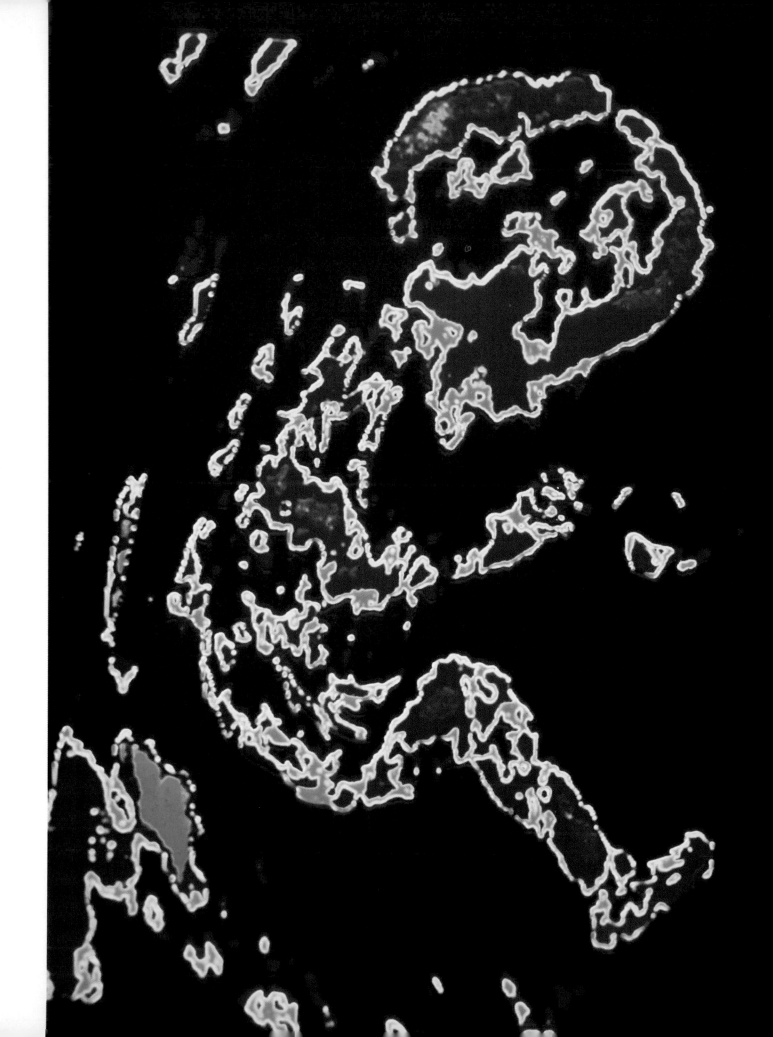

Health in 1968), its application has grown exponentially. The original technology for sound imaging came from Defense Department research in underwater sonar dating back to 1942, and even earlier when airborne radar was developed in the 30's. Today, approximately 7,000 hospitals in the United States have US facilities and over 5 million sonography procedures are done each year. Coupled with the computer, many new applications are being devised.

To generate a US image a transducer (transmitter-receiver) in the shape of a small rod-like (sometimes flat or square) microphone is placed in contact with the surface of the body. A signal of high frequency in the range of 2 to 10 MHz (millions of cycles per second) is transmitted through the skin. The transducer is passed in an arc over the area of the body being investigated. This arc is repeated line after line, until the full width and depth of the area is covered. A scattering occurs when the pulse hits a dense object within the body. A portion of the pulse is then reflected back to the surface of the skin where the transducer now acts as a receiver (microphone). The time delay between sending the pulse and receiving the reflection determines the depth of the target. The size, shape, texture, and location of the target can also be interpreted by variations in the scatter and reflection signals of the original pulse. A picture is displayed on a computer screen almost immediately as the radiologist or technician makes the line-by-line scan.

One of US's great contributions to diagnostic medicine is in the study of human fetal development, where it has provided a mass of new information. Some doctors feel it will be a basis for the development of fetal medicine as a new subspecialty.

A color portrait of a normal fetus before birth by ultrasound. After 25 weeks the radiologist can see the lungs functioning. Sex can often be determined at 15 weeks; blinking, swallowing, and urinating are seen in the third trimester.

Probing painlessly, sonography uses sound waves to look within. The heart of the system is a piezoelectric crystal 1) that converts electric pulses into vibrations that penetrate the body. These sound waves are reflected back to the crystal, which reconverts them into electric signals.

A radiologist or technologist places a transducer containing a crystal 2) on the area to be scanned, such as the abdomen of a pregnant woman. Echoes from the fetus are translated into faint signals, which are processed by a computer into a video imager 3).

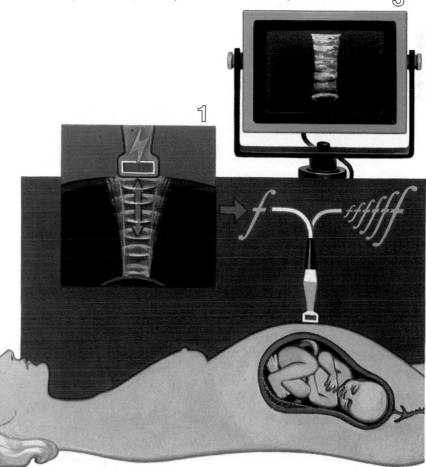

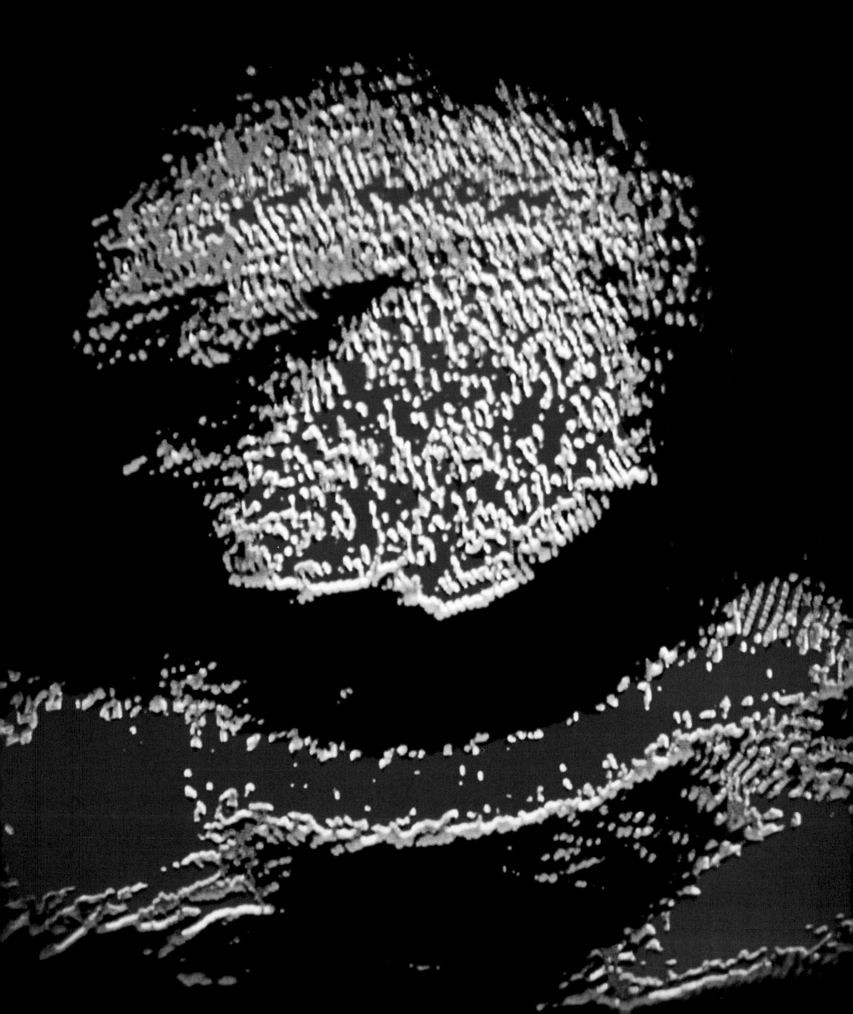

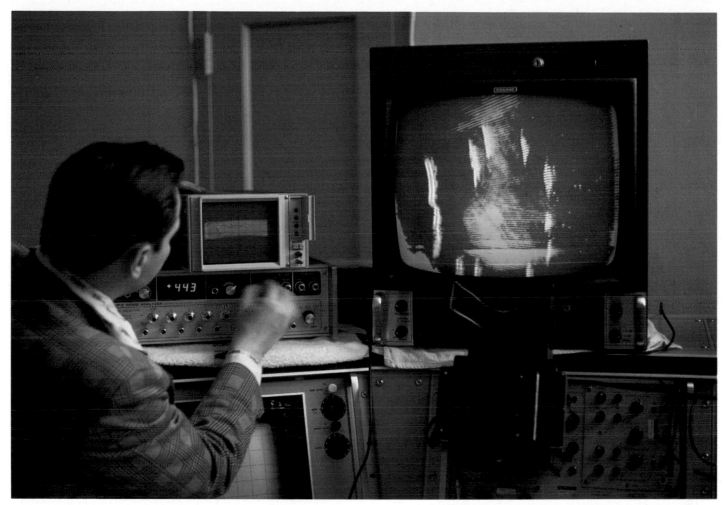

Determining the age of the developing fetus using US is now a standard procedure. Beautiful images can be obtained at five weeks when the fetus is just 5 mm long (even its heartbeat can be detected). Calibrated images can also be obtained over a period of time to analyze growth patterns. The size of the skull, abdomen, and femur shaft can be accurately measured. The exact time when a fetus' lungs are capable of breathing independently can be determined. This information is vital to women in premature labor where early delivery would be fatal to the child.

Fetal weight can be determined by volume measurement and is accurate within 50 grams in birth weights from 500 to 4,000 grams. Growth retardation (a near linear increase in growth should occur after ten weeks) often signals problems.

Fetal anatomy can also be studied and abnormalities such as neural tube brain defects and congenital heart problems can be spotted as early as five months.

Looking inside certain parts of the eye can be a very difficult problem. If a patient's retina, which is sensitive to light, becomes detached from the supporting tissue, blindness may follow. In the past, eye surgeons have often been unable to find what has gone wrong — simply because they had no adequate means of inspection. Now, with the use of ultrasound, they can look into the most delicate parts, even behind the eye, for tumors and other conditions without risk of further damage.

A technologist at the Presbyterian Hospital in New York displays the inside of the human eye on his color monitor. The incredible picture (left) shows a hemorrhage within the eye.

Discoveries like these have resulted in a whole new field of prenatal and neonatal surgery. Ultrasound-guided procedures such as the administering of medication by injection to the fetus, and drainage of excessive fluids by needle aspiration (withdrawal by suction) have become acceptable and almost routine.

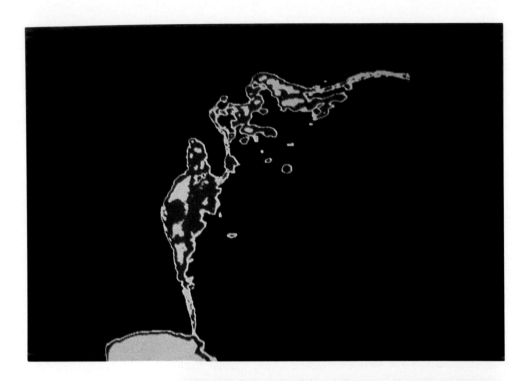

In trouble before birth, Joseph Ward was found to have a tumor growing in his throat that forced him to keep his mouth open inside the womb. Another sonogram displays a cross section of cheeks and rounded tongue, as seen from above, with the tumor, at bottom of image behind the tongue, pushing the tongue forward. Alarmed by the obstruction, Dr. Jason Birnholz of Rush-Presbyterian St. Luke's Medical Center in Chicago asked a surgical team to stand by at Joseph's birth. When the baby failed to breathe, the team opened his breathing passage and saved his life. The obstruction was later removed, and Joseph, now almost three years old (right) has gone on to bigger things.

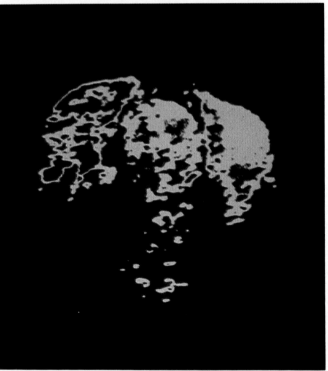

One of the stalwarts in US, first at Massachusetts General Hospital in Boston and now at Rush-Presbyterian-St. Luke's Medical Center in Chicago, is Dr. Jason Birnholz. He performed his first US exam at Georgetown University Hospital in Washington, D.C. in 1968. Dr. Birnholz bubbles with excitement over his new discoveries and their latest applications. He explains: "I can see the lacework of fibers, how an organ is structured, or the elasticity of tissue. I can see a firm liver vs. a floppy or water-logged liver. The presence of collagen, a protein found in the ligaments which has unique reflective properties, determines elasticity. The amount of elasticity can be directly related to disease. I can look at fat: fat content is important in diagnosis of liver disease, in cirrhosis, leukemia, and tumors."

Dr. Birnholz told me of a recent case where the use of US saved a life.

A young school teacher in her 30th week of pregnancy came to the hospital for a routine US scan. Dr. Birnholz noticed that the mother's abdomen was much larger than it should have been and that there was excessive fluid around the baby. On the US scan he saw that the baby's mouth was wide open, that the mouth never changed position, and that the tongue was stretched far forward. Close investigation disclosed a large tumor growing in the throat and neck just under the jaw. A fetus actually begins to swallow after 16 weeks, and the tumor was preventing this.

Dr. Birnholz relayed his findings and films to a pediatric surgeon at St. Luke's Hospital, Dr. Lauren Holinger, who stood by with a surgical team as the baby was delivered. At birth the baby turned blue and was near death. It couldn't breath, the tumor clogging the air passages to the lungs. Immediate action by the surgical team opened the windpipe, and later the tumor was removed.

Today that child, Joseph Ward, is a happy, healthy boy whose life was saved because of the diagnosis achieved through US.

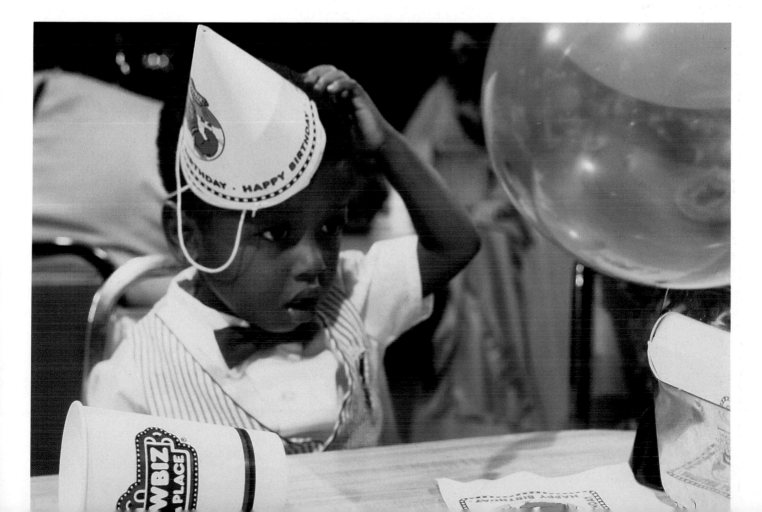

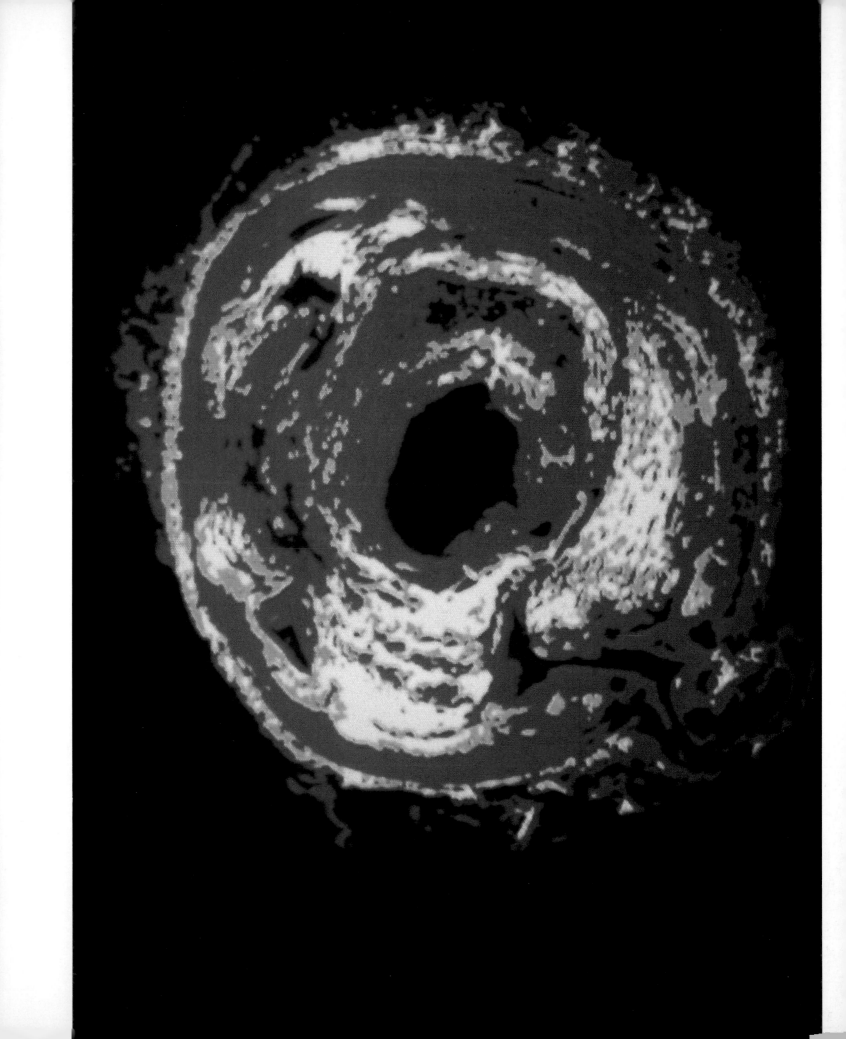

As in Joseph Ward's case, US's great value is that it emits no ionizing radiation and—unlike CT—can be used on pregnant patients. It images soft tissue densities and discriminates them well, detects tumors and lesions, gallstones and kidney stones, images the flow of blood in the major arteries, and is the modality of choice in examining the prostate gland for a possibility of cancer.

Ultrasound is also routinely used in brain surgery. A portable US unit is taken into the operating room, and after the skull is opened the transducer is placed in contact with the brain to locate the tumor (sound will not pass through bone). As reported in Chapter I, some tumors cannot be seen by even the most experienced neurosurgeons. It is imperative that only diseased tissue be removed, otherwise, brain damage could occur. It is equally important that all of the tumor be removed; if not, the tumor could grow back and repeat surgery would be required. The US scan can provide an accurate view, to a resolution of about one 1 mm, of a tumor's position and size.

A new acquisition of the sonographer is digital color Doppler. Assisted by a computer, Doppler shows in picture and sound the flow and eddying currents of human blood.

The Doppler effect was first explained by Austrian physicist Christian Johann Doppler in 1842, and refers to the change in the frequency of sound as an object moves in distance and velocity from a given point. If you are transmitting soundwaves through a blood vessel, the way the sound is returned can signify subtle changes in blood flow. For example, if the blood is flowing smoothly, the sound will resemble a smoothly flowing brook or stream; if the surface over which the blood flows is irregular, there will be an irregularity in the sound. One use of Doppler is in diagnosing an embolism or occlusion of an artery in a patient who has had a stroke. Irregular pressures and flow patterns result just as if a rock had broken loose and was disrupting the flow of a stream. Doppler allows the radiologist to see and hear how much irregularity exists or whether the blood is flowing at all.

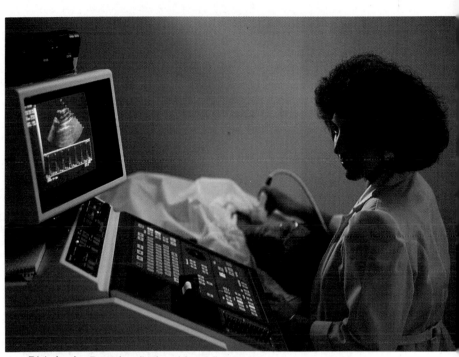

Digital color Doppler displays blood flow in this patient being scanned at a Long Island, New York Imaging Center. The Doppler effect is the shift in frequency of sound waves produced by an object as it moves toward or away from a given point.

This unusual, image-enhanced ultrasound scan is a cross section of a human artery that has been clogged with debris. The lumen (opening) in center is permitting only a small amount of blood to pass through the artery.

Because US is noninvasive, with little or no discomfort to the patient, I was anxious to see and hear how my own arteries were functioning. I visited Dr. Anthony DeMaria, Chief of Cardiology, at the University of Kentucky Hospital in Lexington, and a proponent of cardiac US.

I removed all my clothing from the waist up and lay back on a semireclining bed in a small room. First, Dr. DeMaria applied a thick grease-like salve to my skin over the area of my chest (this assures good contact of the transducer to the skin). Earphones were placed on my head so I would hear the action of my heart. Then, taking the transducer in his right hand and making firm contact with the chest, he moved it in short circular arcs over the skin, just below the ribs. Line by line, in color, my throbbing, pulsing heart was displayed on a small monitor. I could both hear and see the butterfly action of my heart valves, see the oxygen-rich blood eddying up through the ventricles, the oxygen-poor blood eddying down, the flecks and pulses of color swirling and whirling through the heart chambers.

Another expert in US imaging, Dr. Steven Horii at NYU Medical Center, has seen the patient load double from 20 patients a day to 40 patients a day in the eight years he has been doing US. His department examines 5,000 patients a year and uses four scanners. Each of the cases is evaluated by either himself or Dr. B. Nagesh Raghavendra, who heads the department. Dr. Horii told me that patients are scheduled about 45 minutes apart, with an average scan time of 30 minutes. A technician handles the procedure with a radiologist doing the scanning in difficult or serious cases, or when the confirmation of a finding is required.

As we talked, Dr. Horii viewed films brought to him by a technician on the completion of the scans.

Unusual first portrait of a 22-week-old fetus nestled in its mother's womb. The fetus floats and turns endlessly in the liquid that surrounds it in the amniotic sac; sucking its thumb, yawning, blinking, and even urinating.

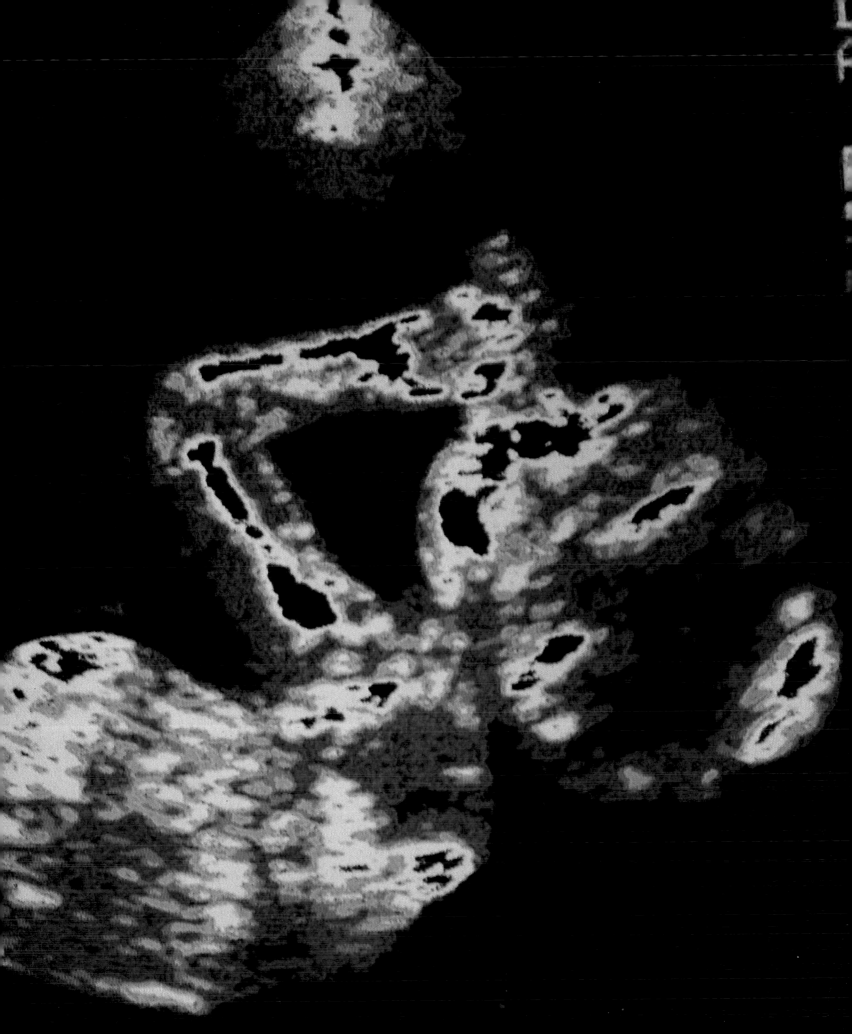

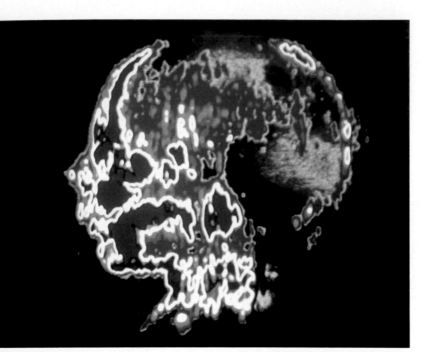

Sagittal (side) view of fully developed fetal head as seen by ultrasound. No biological hazard has yet been discovered from the use of ultrasound in the unborn.

After his evaluation, the patient was released. In one case some indication of a testicular tumor appeared and Horii personally reconfirmed the finding. "You need years of looking at US films to build a mental reference library," commented Dr. Horii. I asked the doctor for cases where his diagnosis had been a life saver and he told me about the case of Mary Masliah.

A life-threatening problem in pregnancy exists when the fertilized ovum begins growing outside the uterine cavity. Called an ectopic pregnancy, very few symptoms exist in the initial stages: light vaginal spotting or light bleeding might be the only warning. But the problem is serious since unpredictable hemorrhage can easily occur very suddenly.

Mary came for a routine scan in her tenth week of pregnancy. Her obstetrician was concerned that her uterus was smaller than it should have been and she was experiencing some slight spotting, but no major pain or discomfort.

Dr. Horii found, on viewing the films, the developing embryo clearly visible at the junction of the right fallopian tube and the uterus. Its continued growth threatened the main uterine artery and a major hemorrhage was certainly possible, if not inevitable. This is called a cornual pregnancy and no other imaging technique could have been used to find it without radiation risk. Mary's pregnancy was terminated surgically.

Dr. Horii sees a great and growing future for US. In the past six months, he has been using transrectal and transvaginal equipment, in which a transducer is placed on the end of a probe and inserted into the rectum or vagina. In each case, by using a higher frequency signal, greater resolution is obtained. Prostate cancer, so common in elderly men, can be determined by a rectal US probe; the vaginal probe assists in early detection of embryonic abnormalities.

Ultrasound diagnosis was a life saver for little William Mahoney of Manlius, New York. His story was told by Dr. Beverly Spirt, a noted radiologist at SUNY Health Sciences Center in Syracuse, and by Will's mother, Mrs. Catherine Mahoney. Mrs. Mahoney was told of the advent of twins in the eighth week of her pregnancy during a routine US examination. William and his sister Greer were born

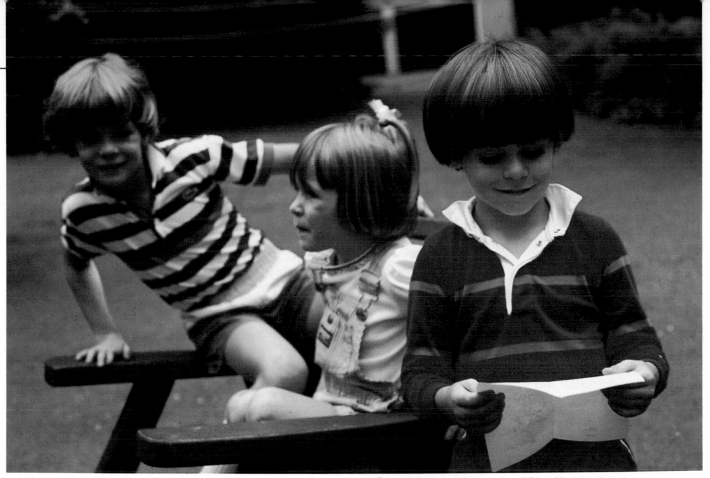

William Mahoney, after years of ill health, benefitted from ultrasound. A faulty kidney duct was detected and replaced restoring him to good health. His brother and sister play behind him at their home in Manlius, New York.

on January 10, 1983; both were normal.

But at about age two, Willy experienced periodic vomiting attacks that grew increasingly worse. Some lasted as long as ten or twelve hours. Initially diagnosed as a "viral attack," the wretching continued and no medication seemed to work. At wits end, Mrs. Mahoney persisted in getting a second and third opinion. A barium GI series of x-rays disclosed nothing. Heart and head studies were negative and brain tumors and epilepsy were ruled out. The attacks continued, one lasting 14 hours.

In desperation, William's father called his cousin, a cardiologist. He recommended a US scan and Mrs. Mahoney contacted Dr. Spirt in nearby Syracuse. A life-threatening kidney malfunction with a serious duct abnormality was discovered (ureteropelvic junction obstruction or UPJO for short), and surgery was performed the next day. A plastic implant was made to replace the faulty ureter junction, and Willy recovered after eight weeks of convalescence. His surgeon now monitors William's left kidney twice a year with US to observe the implant and confirm that the kidney is functioning normally.

Dr. Spirt told me other stories of patients whose lives have been saved or prolonged by an accurate diagnosis based on US images.

A 32-year-old woman with a newly transplanted kidney was suffering from extreme pain. Ultrasound found four large areas of fluid around the kidney. These buildups are common and result from surgical procedures used in transplant operations. The fluid was removed by needle aspiration and the patient is now fine. Ultrasound is also helpful in evaluating transplanted kidney rejection. Another case involved a fetus with excess fluid in the brain (hydrocephalus) which was properly diagnosed before birth. Immediately after birth, a shunt for drainage of the fluid was implanted; the young lad, now three, is thriving.

Fifty percent of US scans are now performed on obstetrical patients, but as new Doppler ultrasound machines come into general use more and more applications will be in the analysis of heart disease

A picture made with ultrasound in the sixth month of pregnancy shows the face of a healthy fetus with mouth open in a yawn. ``By this point the fetus does just about everything it will do after birth,'' said Dr. Christopher Merritt of New Orleans, who obtained the image. ``It yawns, blinks, and even sucks it thumb.'' Sonography lets us share these sneak previews by beaming high-frequency sound waves into the womb in short pulses. A computer translates the echoes that bounce back into an image of the fetus. The only body-scanning technique recommended for pregnant women, sonography is also well suited for examinations of the breasts, heart, liver, and gall bladder.

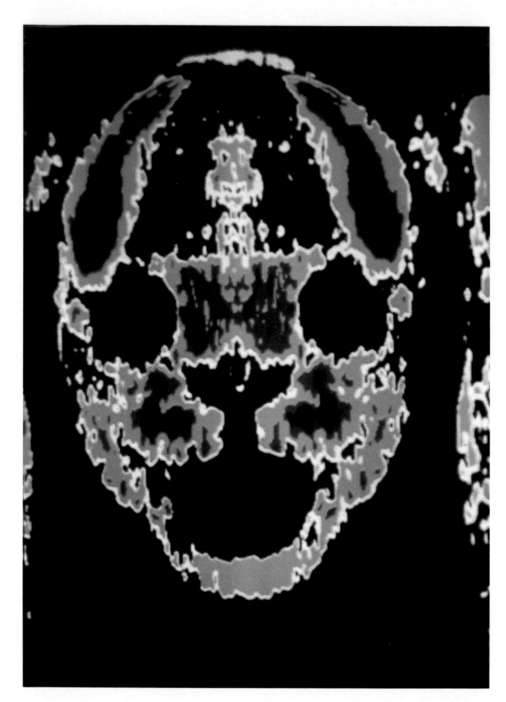

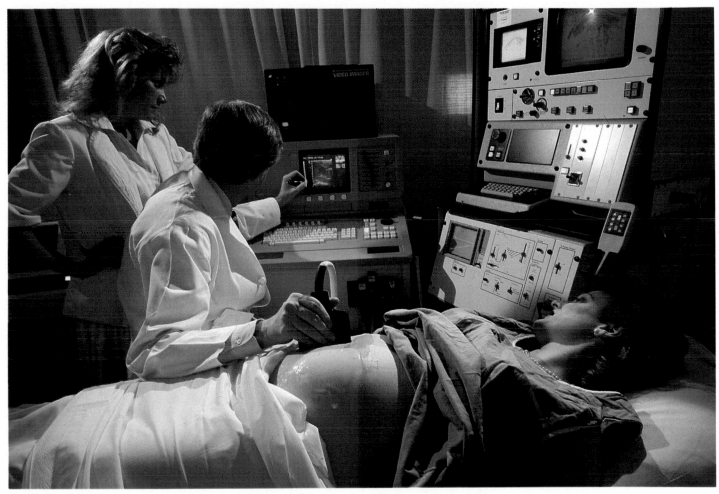

Dr. Christopher Merritt at the console of the scanner obtaining pictures of a yawning fetus (left).

and heart function. Dr. Christopher Merritt at the Ochsner Clinic in New Orleans looks for Doppler to be used in observing the blood flow in all parts of the body. He sees the possibility of early cancer detection. "Cancer induces the formation of new blood vessels which are not normal. We will look at the tissues that are supplied by these blood vessels which may be some of the earliest changes we can perceive."

During our visit, Dr. Merritt proceeded with a routine scan of a young mother in her 28th week of pregnancy. She was thrilled as we watched the fetus kick and turn, suck its thumb, seem to cross its legs, and finally give a huge yawn. Only about half of the parents want to know the sex of their child which

can often be determined as early as 15 weeks (males earlier). But, of course, all of them want that first Polaroid snapshot of the TV screen showing the fetus in utero. That psychological process, called bonding, now begins before the child's birth.

With all the joy these few moments held for the child's mother, Dr. Merritt and myself, Dr. Merritt had a much sadder duty to perform that afternoon. As I readied to leave, I found him seated in a small side office consoling a sobbing expectant mother. The US scan had determined that the child she was carrying had died. There was no movement, no heartbeat, no sign of life of any kind, only a silent motionless form on the flickering screen, hands over its head, knees tucked under its chin, asleep forever.

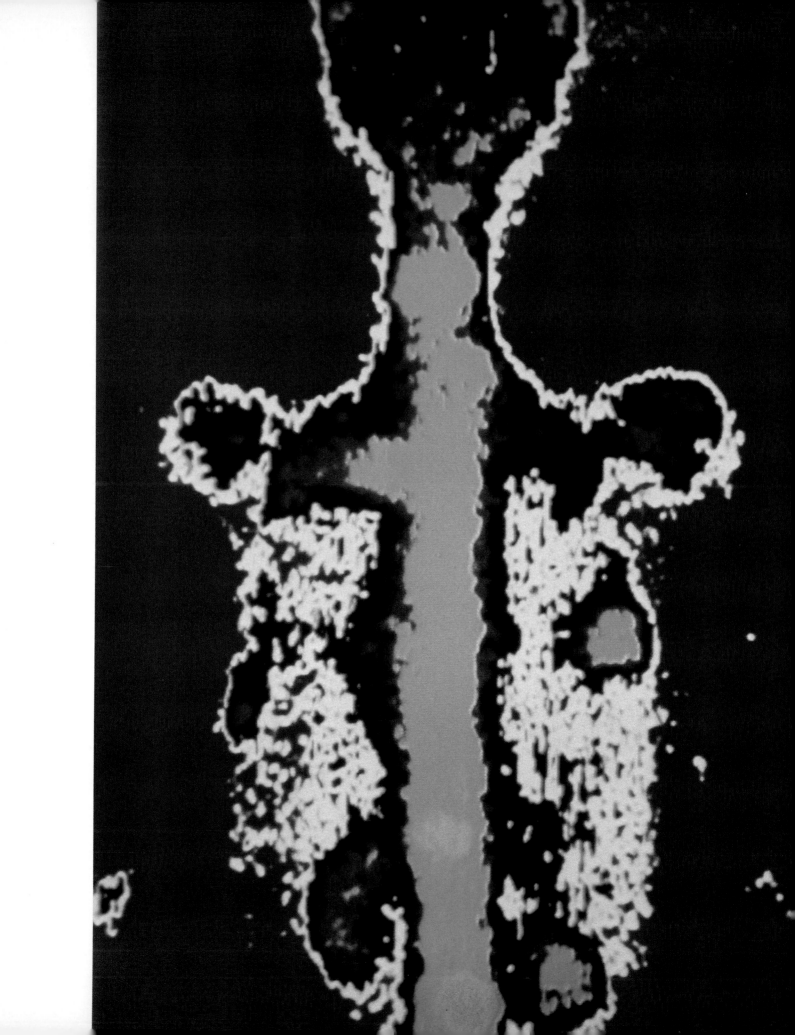

IV. NUCLEAR MEDICINE

"Detect and prevent"

"Howard, there may be something wrong with your heart." Addressing me was Dr. K. Lance Gould who heads the Positron Diagnostic and Research Center at the University of Texas Medical School in Houston. He had agreed to scan my heart using a PET (positron emission tomography) scanner. The ground rules were that I would write about the test only if the results were normal. Otherwise, my health might be compromised by the rigors of pursuing the story. I had taken the gamble and, apparently, lost.

Dr. Gould told me that he had received my medical records the night before and that my EKG (electrocardiogram) showed a potential problem. "You may not be able to write this story," he explained. "This story," as he called it, had suddenly become deadly serious. I was subjecting my beyond-middle-age body to the scrutiny of a machine that could detect coronary disease in its earliest stages. We decided to proceed with the test and worry about the story after the results were in.

Minutes earlier head research nurse Mary Haynie had used a fluoroscope to obtain an image of my heart and outline its position on my chest with a magic marker. I lay faceup on a table and was slowly moved into the $1.6 million PET scanner—a huge, two-ton metallic doughnut with a center hole just large enough for me to squeeze through.

As a young cardiologist, Dr. Gould had questioned the conventional medical practice of dealing with coronary disease only after complications had occurred; his early laboratory

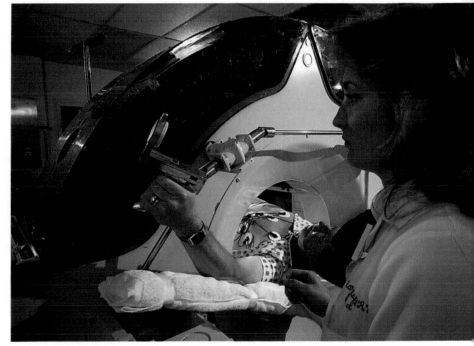

In the doughnut hole of a PET scanner, a patient squeezes a hand grip that helps stimulate the heart during a stress test. The PET scanner, at the University of Texas in Houston, images trace amounts of radioisotopes in the heart to determine whether or not muscle tissues are receiving an adequate supply of blood. Electrodes on the chest record an electrocardiogram which is monitored by research nurse Mary Haynie.

A bone scan creates a picture of the skeleton that often reveals abnormalities much earlier than conventional radiographs.

work indicated that coronary disease could be detected much sooner. "If you could screen for coronary disease and find it five or ten years in advance of trouble—if that could be done—you could save countless lives."

Today, running a center with a staff of 75, he uses nuclear medicine screening techniques to identify coronary disease even in patients without symptoms. And for this I was a prime candidate: a tense, overweight, hard-driven Type A personality, pushing past 60.

Mary Haynie's fluoroscopy showed that my heart, unlike most others, did not "hang vertically" in the chest cavity but was tipped sideways. Since the scanner covers only 11 cm (about 4½"), the position of my body in the doughnut was critical. I remained perfectly still for 20 minutes while the scanner collected data.

Mary and a technologist injected a low-level radioactive tracer (in this case N-13 ammonia) through the intravenous catheter in my right arm. Freshly brewed by Dr.Gould's cyclotron, the tracer had a ten-minute half-life (the time it takes to lose half of its radioactivity), so it had to be administered quickly and with precision.

Fifteen minutes of scan time elapsed while my heart beat normally and I lay quietly. I heard only the hum of the scanner's cooling fans and the beeping of the EKG machine that monitored me continuously. I experienced some anxiety; Mary and Dr. Gould hovered about—observing, checking, recording data.

Next, it was time to check my heart's response to stress. Dipyridamole, a drug that simulates stress to the heart, was injected through the intravenous catheter that had remained in place. Mary then gave me a hand grip to flex the finger, wrist, and forearm muscles; I clenched it tightly until the gauge recorded a pressure of 20 pounds. This, Mary explained, would increase blood flow to the heart even more than a conventional treadmill test.

A second injection of the N-13 nuclear tracer entered my arm, and the scanner studied my heart under stress for an additional 15 minutes. The "dipy" as the team called it, taxed my stamina, and my face took on a red flush. My left arm shivered a bit as I maintained 20 pounds of pressure on the hand grip, the EKG continually sounding its beep, beep, beep.

To break the monotony I talked to Mary about her family and mine. Her father had died of a heart attack at age 47 (mine had died of a heart attack at age 86), and her mother was left alone to raise her and seven brothers and sisters. Perhaps, I thought, the test I was undergoing could have warned her father of his peril.

The exhausting 15 minutes finally passed, the humming of the scanner stopped, Mary removed the catheter from my right arm, and I released the grip in my left hand. After an hour and a half of lying still, it was over.

"Will I glow in the dark?" I asked Mary as I got up off the table.

As in the other modalities covered in this book, the computer had been the key in developing nuclear medicine technology, and the PET computer processed a staggering amount of information as we waited for the data to assume picture form, in color, on the monitor. Now came the moment of truth.

First the monitor showed my heart beating normally with the blood supply circulating through the heart muscle. The monitor flashed again, and alongside the first image appeared a picture of my heart under stress. Transfixed, we all studied the two images: if they should differ, it would indicate a blood supply problem and signal the death of my story on nuclear medicine, but the images matched perfectly: Dr. Gould smiled, Mary smiled, I smiled.

What had caused Dr. Gould's original concern? "Because your heart lies on its side instead of hanging normally," he explained, "the EKGs in your medical records were misleading. Not until we obtained the PET image to confirm the heart's position and flow capacity did I find all was okay. You have a healthy heart. You can write your story. Come back again in two years."

I had no aftereffects from my PET scan but experienced a headache after leaving the center. It may have been because, as directed, I had missed my usual hearty breakfast. And, of course, I didn't glow in the dark!

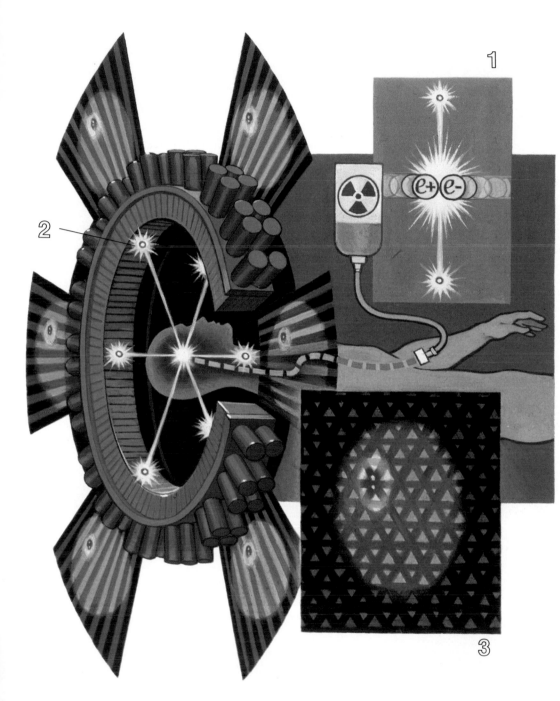

1

2

3

To spy on the brain in action, PET scanners watch the way brain cells consume substances such as sugar. The substance is tagged with a radioisotope brewed in a small, low-energy cyclotron. The isotope has a short half-life, meaning that it loses half of its radioactivity within only minutes or hours of being created. Injected into the body, the radioactive solution emits positrons wherever it flows. The positrons collide with electrons, and the two annihilate one another, releasing a burst of energy in the form of two gamma rays. These rays shoot in opposite directions (1) and strike crystals in a ring of detectors (2) around the patient's head, causing the crystals to light up. A computer records the location of each flash and plots the source of radiation, translating that data into an image (3).

By tracing the radioactive substance, the radiologist can pinpoint areas of abnormal brain activity or determine the health of cells.

Unlike PET, which generally requires a cyclotron on site, SPECT uses commercially available radioisotopes, greatly reducing the costs of the procedure.

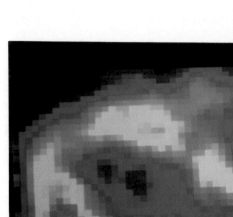

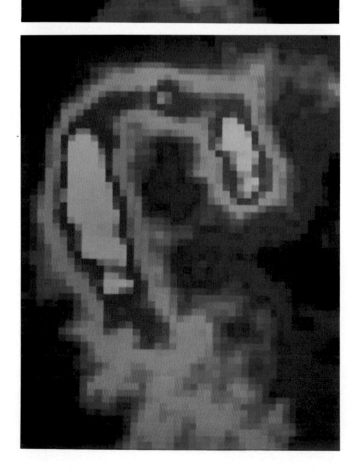

The PET scan is but one of several nuclear imaging techniques. All use a similar procedure in which a radioactive tracer (there are many) is injected, swallowed, or inhaled. It mixes with its analogue (blood is one) and follows the same pathway. When the atoms of the tracer decay, they emit photons. The distribution of the tracer in the patient is imaged by recording this photon emission using scintillation or gamma cameras.

Throughout my travels in preparing this book, I have often been amazed at how fate, luck, or persistence have been factors in ultimately saving a life. Fate certainly took a hand when Dr. Charles C. Douglass, a Houston oncologist, heard about a lecture on PET at the University of Texas Medical School. Dr. Richard Goldstein, an associate of Dr. Gould, frequently lectures on PET to inform both his peers and the general public about preventive coronary care. Dr. Douglass told me his story.

"A doctor specializing in cancer therapy has lots of problems" he began. "On call seven days a week, 24 hours a day, I felt like I was on a merry-go-round. I lost control of my life; my practice ran me. Many

Glowing brightly on a video screen, a PET image shows a normal blood supply in a heart without stress (bottom). White, orange, and yellow areas show the walls of the left ventricle — as seen from above — absorbing a radioisotope, N-13 ammonia, from the blood. Both PET and SPECT depict the distribution of blood in tissue, but PET does so with greater accuracy.

A second PET image shows the same heart under stress (top) and reveals a problem in the blood supply to the ventricular wall in the upper half of the picture. Stress was induced by an injection of dipyridamole, which simulates exercise by boosting blood flow to healthy muscle tissues. The increased flow, however, is blocked by an artery with a constriction.

In the unstressed heart the scanner shows white and orange where absorption of the radioisotope is greatest. But in the heart under stress there is only yellow in its upper half, indicating a partial blockage in the coronary artery feeding that part of the heart. Left untreated, this defect may eventually cause a heart attack. Detected by the PET scanner, it could be prevented.

people in our society have lost control of their lives—I was one of them. I stayed in the rat race, and didn't see the damage that was being done to me. I felt lousy. I would walk six blocks and get chest pains. Worried, I called my friend Dr. Abdul Ali, a cardiologist.'' Dr. Ali had also heard Dr. Goldstein's lecture and recommended a stress test. ''The next day, on Saturday, I took a stress test which was negative, but I did have a little pain during the last two minutes.''

Armed with the information from Goldstein's lecture, Dr. Douglass decided to undergo a PET scan and was scheduled for Tuesday. ''I remembered saying to myself 'I don't want to be a cardiac cripple','' Dr. Douglass told me.

Dr. Gould's scanner clearly indicated trouble (a 90% occlusion in the left anterior artery was later diagnosed).

''The pain worsened over the weekend, so the following Monday I met Dr. Ali in the Emergency Room. Based on the information confirmed by Dr. Gould and the PET scan, I decided on angioplasty. A first effort on Tuesday was to dissolve a blood clot in the left anterior descending artery just past the first perforator. Awake during the procedure, I wanted the clot dissolved to be able to dodge a real bullet: bypass surgery. The clot wouldn't dissolve, so on Thursday I went back to the cath lab. I would have done anything to prevent surgery. They spent another three hours trying to get a catheter into the artery but couldn't make it. The following Wednesday I went in for a single bypass.''

Today Dr. Douglass is fine and is an enthusiastic booster for PET. It is certainly possible that if alerted earlier by a PET scan, his bypass surgery could have been prevented.

''Stress contributed to my problem,'' he maintains. ''In a subspecialty practice like mine, you must be available to go anywhere at any time. If you

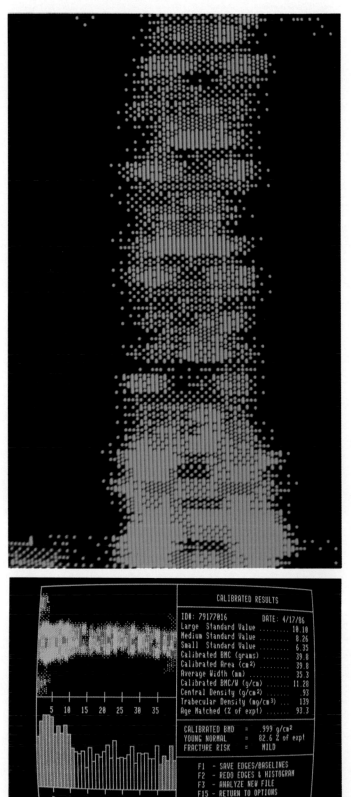

Checking for bone density loss in postmenopausal women, a spinal bone scan can reveal the possible risk of fractures. The monitor indicates only minor risk in this patient. Screening for osteoporosis in women older than 51 years uses this nuclear medicine technique.

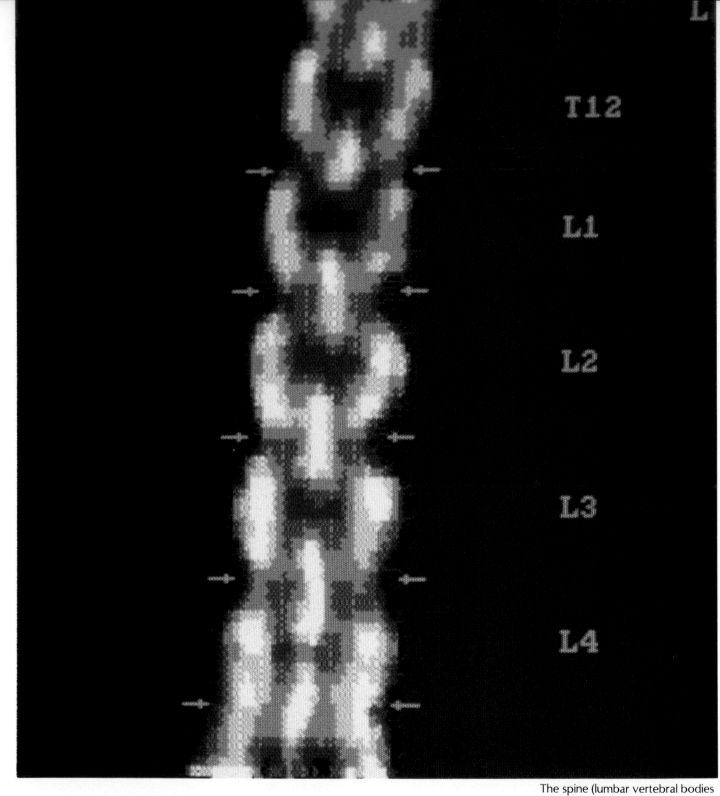

T12

L1

L2

L3

L4

The spine (lumbar vertebral bodies L1–L5) as viewed by dual-photon absorptiometry. Bone mineral or calcium content is precisely measured by an external noninvasive technique. Osteoporosis, or bone mineral loss, affects one in every four women after menopause.

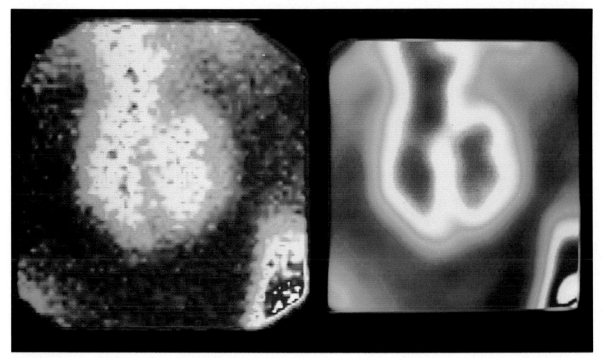

Gamma camera scan of the heart is used to check blood
volume and wall muscle action in this cardiac patient.

don't, you won't have a practice. Why have bypass
surgery if you can prevent it."

In December of 1987 at the annual meeting of
the Radiological Society of North America in
Chicago, I met with Dr. Philip O. Alderson, a
specialist in nuclear medicine, and director of the
department at Columbia Presbyterian Hospital in
New York. His work at the hospital falls into four
categories.

"The most common procedure in the
department is a full-body bone scan done with a
single plane gamma camera using technetium 99m
tagged to phosphonates as the radionuclide tracer.
Once injected, it travels to and is absorbed by the
bones of the entire skeleton. The gamma camera
measures the radiation and forms an image on film.
By looking at spots of increased or decreased
absorption of the tracer, defects and problems can
be identified."

Dr. Alderson feels that this is the procedure of
choice to detect metastatic bone disease (spread of
a cancer from one place to another) in many cases.

The second most common application of

nuclear medicine is in the use of electrocardiographic
multiple gated acquisition (MUGA) for imaging the
heart. In this procedure, using technetium-tagged red
blood cells, a study of the heart's muscular wall motion
is possible as well as a study of the heart's chambers.

The third application is the thallium scan. Here
the radioactive thallium is injected and areas of the
heart receiving insufficient blood and oxygen will
show less thallium uptake than healthy tissue. Areas
of heart muscle being deprived of blood and oxygen
are evidence of heart disease.

Lungs are viewed in the fourth most frequent
application of nuclear medicine. The radiologist in
this case is looking for a pulmonary embolism (a clot
in the lung's blood supply). Ten percent of cases of
pulmonary embolism are fatal, so quick detection
and therapy are usually of urgent concern.
Technetium is again the tracer of choice because it
attaches to particles of albumin that adhere
temporarily to normal lung tissue, allowing an image
to be recorded. Here again, an injection in the veins
followed by a gamma camera scan reveals the
embolus. This technique (called a perfusion scan)

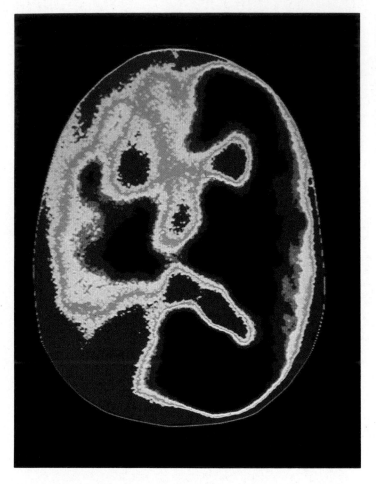

Gaining strength every day, 2-year-old Ryan Petersen of Great Falls, Virginia was given little chance of surviving childhood. Unable to find a cause for the seizures he had suffered since birth, his doctors had given Ryan's parents little hope. Then, while Ryan was visiting his grandparents in southern California, his seizures worsened. His parents took him to the UCLA Medical Center where a PET scan (left) showed normal activity in the right hemisphere of his brain but only minimal activity in his left. After surgery to remove most of the left hemisphere, Ryan works with physical therapist Francie Mitchell (right) to improve control of his muscles.

UCLA Medical Center. Blond, blue-eyed Ryan Petersen was born on September 23, 1984. After only eight hours of life he suffered his first seizure which lasted just one minute and was diagnosed at the time as tonic-clonic unilateral spasms. At three months of age the problem increased with spasms as frequent as five times daily. Again, a frantic mother tried every possible course of action. A CT scan showed nothing. A new drug (nitrazapam) was tried, worked for a few weeks, then proved ineffective. Mrs. Petersen was told that nothing more could be done for her son.

Expecting that Ryan could not survive much longer, Mrs. Petersen decided on a Christmas visit to California to see Ryan's grandparents. After two days in Los Angeles, the boy's health deteriorated even more—the seizures now lasting from 30 to 40 minutes.

Desperate, Mrs. Petersen took Ryan to UCLA Medical Center where Dr. Harry Chungani, pediatric neurologist, ordered a PET scan. It revealed that almost the entire left side of Ryan's brain was inactive.

Surgery was performed at UCLA by noted brain surgeon, Dr. Warwick Peacock, who performed similar operations in South Africa and had just recently arrived in the United States. After a four-month recuperation in California, Ryan returned home to Great Falls, Virginia. He has not had a single seizure since surgery and attends physical therapy sessions to improve muscle functions. His case is being closely studied, and it is possible that the right brain may, in time, take on many of the functions that it previously shared with the left brain.

may be preceded by a ventilation scan. In this case, a radioactive gas is mixed with oxygen which is inhaled through a mask. The camera makes a picture after the first breath; more pictures are obtained after several minutes of inhaling and after the gas mixture has been exhaled and the patient is breathing room air. Embolism, pneumonia, asthma, bronchitis, emphysema and even cancer can be diagnosed by perfusion and ventilation scans. Radiation here is again at a very low level.

Dr. Alderson described the radiation level (equal to a chest x-ray) as "a ten-pound bag dropped on a rabbit. Drop the bag and you kill him, but a dribble of sand from the bag does no harm at all."

A wonderful success story involving the use of PET in diagnosis was told to me by Dr. Michael Phelps in the Department of Nuclear Medicine,

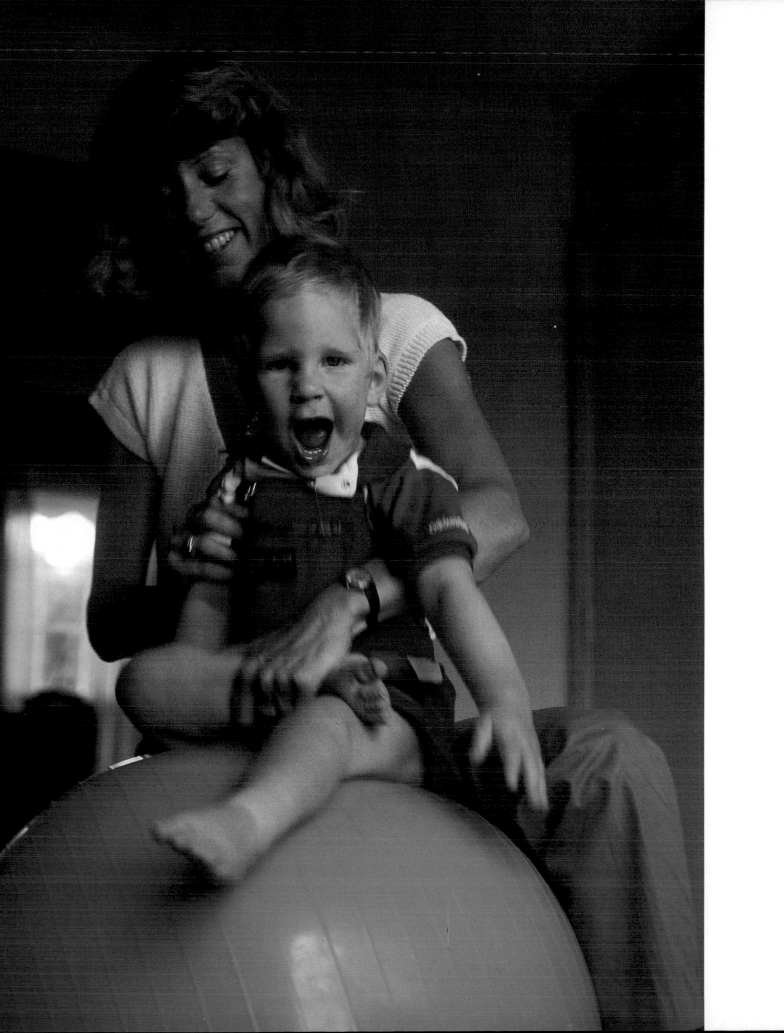

A distinguished radiologist, Dr. John McAfee, Director of Radiological Science and Research in Diagnostic Radiology at SUNY Health Sciences Center in Syracuse, New York, has spent over 30 years of his career in nuclear medicine. His research efforts center on finding the best tracers to be used in nuclear imaging, what has least risk to the patient, and what gives the best spatial resolution. Probably of most importance is his study of radiolabeled monoclonal antibodies that will help in both detection of disease and drug delivery to specific problem areas.

Besides the conventionally used tracers—thallium for the heart, and technetium compounds for the liver, bones, lungs, and kidneys—many new chemicals are being discovered. He told me about ceretec (now widely used in Europe) that localizes in the brain, and a new material called RP-30 that localizes in heart muscle. "With another new agent (indium oxine) approved for use in 1986, we can tell just where the white blood cells are fighting infection."

In Switzerland, a new monoclonal antibody (MoAb 47) labels white cells spontaneously, greatly shortening the previous procedure which required separating red and white cells in the laboratory. With added knowledge about the white cells, quicker, more effective treatment is possible.

Dr. McAfee voiced "frustration" with the Food and Drug Administration's regulatory procedures. Only a few of the many new drug applications have been approved since 1982, but he remains excited by the prospects of the development of new drugs that "fool mother nature." Several radioactive proteins attach themselves to blood clots (fibrin) so that they can be detected by the gamma camera.

Picture of confusion. An image obtained using single photon emission computed tomography (SPECT) shows a patch of darkness in the brain of a 57-year-old man. Reflecting a decrease in blood flow to the parietal lobes — where sensations from the eyes and ears are associated with memory — darkness symbolizes the agony of Alzheimer's disease.

SPECT shows blood flow by imaging trace amounts of radioisotopes. A more versatile technique, positron emission tomography (PET), can also measure metabolism, revealing how well the body is working. The use of radioactive tracers is well suited to studies of epilepsy, schizophrenia, Parkinson's disease, and stroke.

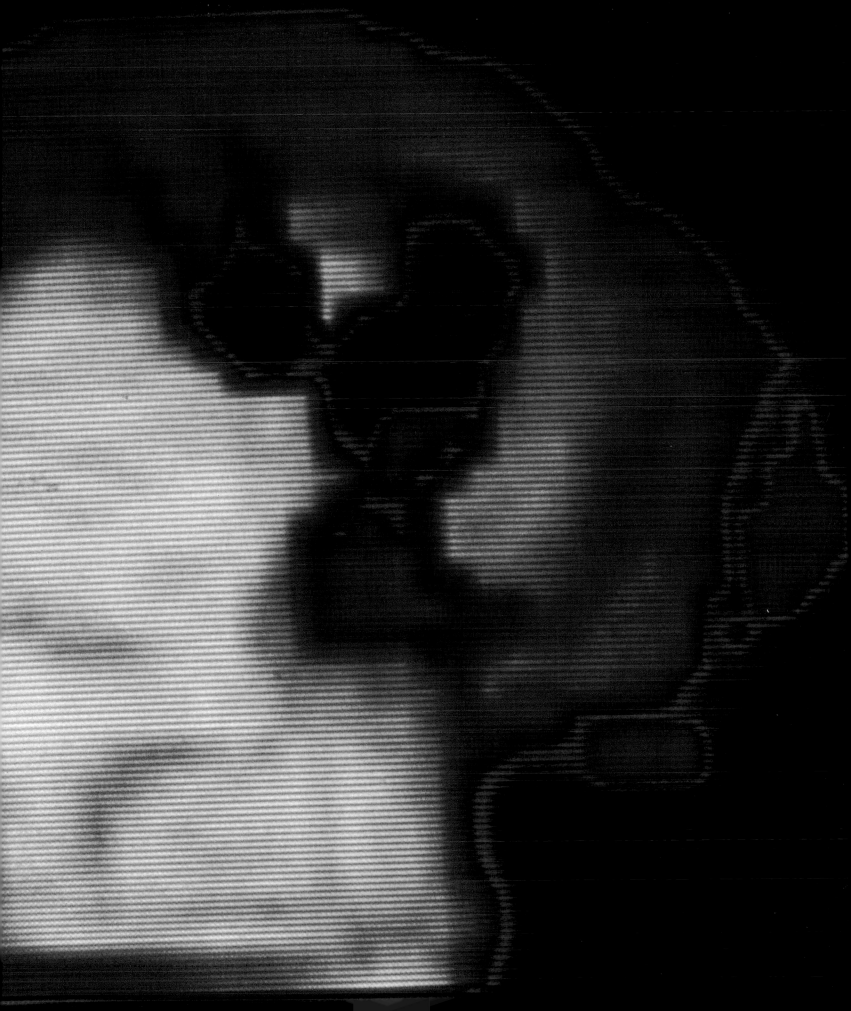

The whole body is captured in a bone scan obtained using radioisotope tracers. Created by a gamma camera, the image depicts emissions of gamma rays from a phosphate tagged with technetium-99m, a low-level radioactive material. Injected into the blood stream, the phosphate comes to rest mainly in bones, producing a comprehensive view of the skeletal system. This study was done to determine whether or not cancer had spread to the bones from a tumor in the breast of a 56-year-old woman. It had not.

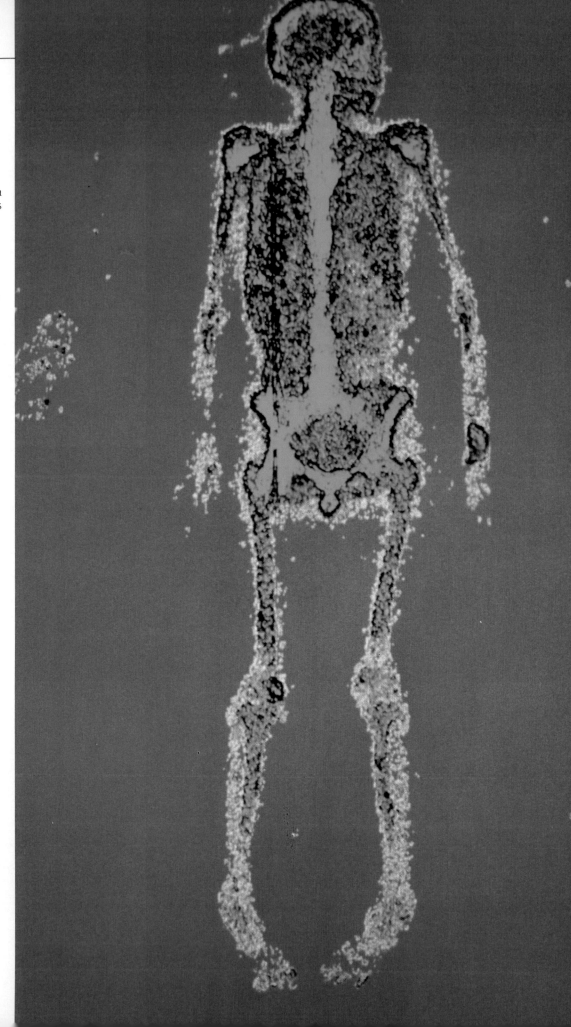

Other proteins can be labeled with radioactivity, providing new knowledge about their organ distribution and function.

Another eminent radiologist, Dr. B. Leonard Holman, Chairman, Department of Radiology at Brigham and Women's Hospital in Boston, Massachusetts, and his technologist, Bob English, have used SPECT to achieve accurate three-dimensional diagnostic images of Alzheimer's disease. "We are equally interested in the absorption or lack of absorption of the radionuclide tracer. SPECT is our screening technique and is a simple and painless procedure for the patient," Dr. Holman told me. The radioactive material is injected intravenously, and a waiting time of about an hour is required until it is absorbed (this varies according to the specific isotope and organ being studied). Then the patient lies still while the camera rotates the body. There are no aftereffects.

Dr. Holman sees great opportunity in studying the chemistry of the brain with information provided by monoclonal antibodies, and receptors of the neurotransmitters and neuroreceivers in psychiatric disease. Simply stated, a radionuclide tracer is piggybacked on a monoclonal antibody. The monoclonal antibody makes a beeline to an antigen or disease fighter in the organ under attack. Detection of "what" and "where" is then possible. Dr. Holman shares Dr. McAfee's frustration with the FDA.

Just as Dr. Horii (Chapter III) is using probes in his ultrasound work, Dr. Jim Woolfenden at the University of Arizona Health Science Center in Tucson is developing new radiation detector probes. The detectors are not unlike those of the gamma camera, SPECT, or PET, but differ because they are miniaturized and are inserted into a body cavity via a snake-like cable that carries the detector as close as possible to the organ being studied. The latest detectors are only 2 mm in diameter (about 5/64") and the hand-held probe is only 1 cm in diameter (less than 1/2"). A picture can thus be obtained from inside the body!

Dr. Woolfenden concentrates on researching the spread of cancers to the lymphatic system. His inventory of radiotracers can monitor blood flow

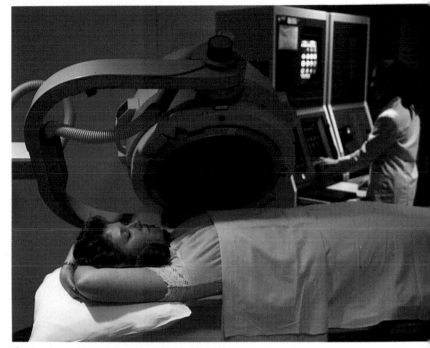

The basic tool in nuclear medicine is the gamma camera. It is used to scan the brain, thyroid gland, lungs, heart, liver, gallbladder and bones.

and volume, and oxygen, glucose, and protein metabolism. These probes can literally take the detector to the tumor. They show promise in the detection of prostate cancer.

Dr. Woolfenden has also developed another probe made up of layers of semiconductors and radiation detectors that "look out" at different angles. The probe is inserted in the esophagus; several levels of data are generated as the probe is withdrawn.

After talking with Dr. Woolfenden, it is apparent that the technology boom of the past 20 years will be dwarfed by advances in the next 20 years.

Dr. Naomi Alazraki, a distinguished radiologist working at Emory University Hospital in Atlanta, Georgia, is another pioneer in the development of new applications of nuclear medicine. She traced for me the development of nuclear medicine from the first PET scans of the 1960s to the gamma camera of the 70s and finally SPECT of the 80s.

"Nuclear medicine was the first medical specialty to use the computer," Dr. Alazraki told me.

"The computer made it possible to acquire and analyze quantitative data on organ function quickly."

Working with Dr. Ernie Garcia and collaborators at Georgia Tech, Dr. Alazraki and the radiology team at Emory have developed a novel computer imaging technique called the bull's-eye plot which is used to evaluate SPECT scans. Here the image appears on the computer screen as if the heart were set on a base and compressed or collapsed to resemble a pie. The pie is divided into 32 sectors resembling a dartboard or marksman's target thus creating a kind of "heart map." In most cases, we are looking at the muscular tissue of the heart (myocardium) and its ability to function normally as indicated by the amount of the blood supply. Where the blood supply is poor the uptake of the radioisotope is poor, and the area is shown in a different color on the viewing screen. As little as 1% deviation from normal blood supply is registered by the bull's-eye image. A change of less than 1% is white, followed by yellow, red, dark blue, light blue, and finally black. Black areas indicate a variance of over 7% from the norm and usually indicate a degree of coronary artery disease or at worst an infarct.

I sat with Dr. Alazraki one afternoon in her viewing room as she examined the SPECT-bull's-eye scans of her patients. She was surrounded by eager resident doctors in radiology, mainly women. We watched as multiple images—obtained just hours or minutes earlier—danced on the computer screens. First were cardiac images of a middle-aged man, recorded while under stress, showing three black areas in the periphery of the bull's-eye image. The non-stress images indicated no abnormality. The diagnosis: coronary occlusion. Next were images of a man who had undergone angioplasty six months previously to "open" an artery. This latest scan showed that the same major artery was closing up again (narrowing or stenosing). Dr. Alazraki explained that this is common in about one-quarter to one-third of angioplasty patients. In addition, another black area evidenced itself in the bull's-eye pie cut in the lower left quadrant. This patient would have to return for angioplasty or bypass surgery.

Some of the patients scanned showed no abnormality and got a clean bill of health, much as I had been given after my PET scan. It struck me that the SPECT-bull's-eye method might be a quick, easy means of predicting heart attacks long before they happen, just as Dr. Gould is doing with his PET scans in Houston.

In similar work at Emory, magnetic resonance images of the heart and other parts of the anatomy are being viewed in "bullet" projections that are displayed in color, with any abnormalities appearing as black, crater-like areas.

So far in this chapter we have restricted our explanation to the imaging of radiation emitted from radioactive compounds that are injected, swallowed or inhaled. But there is another new method of imaging based on an external source of radiation. Dr. David F. Preston at the Department of Nuclear Medicine, University of Kansas Medical Center in Kansas City, explained it to me.

"A source of radioactive gadolinium (Gd) is housed in a shielded container beneath the patient who lies prone on a special pallet. A narrow beam emitted from the source travels up through the patient into a detector above. The source and detector move together, mechanically scanning the patient's lower spine or hips."

The procedure is called dual photon absorptiometry (DPA). Using this method, mineral (calcium) content of bone is measured precisely. A low calcium content is usually due to osteoporosis (softening of bone), increasing the risk of fractures in the spine or hips. This new DPA method is becoming popular because one of every four post-menopausal women suffers from severe bone loss due to osteoporosis.

Dr. Preston explained to me that two photons are emitted from the same isotope, hence the term "dual" in the name "DPA." A source of gadolinium will last for a whole year; the scan is fast, efficient, and relatively inexpensive.

"Nuclear medicine can find disease before there are anatomical changes," Dr. Preston explained. "Our aim is early detection so we can direct a management regimen to prevent bone deterioration. We might even avert the development of osteoporosis by a preventive program that begins in adolescence."

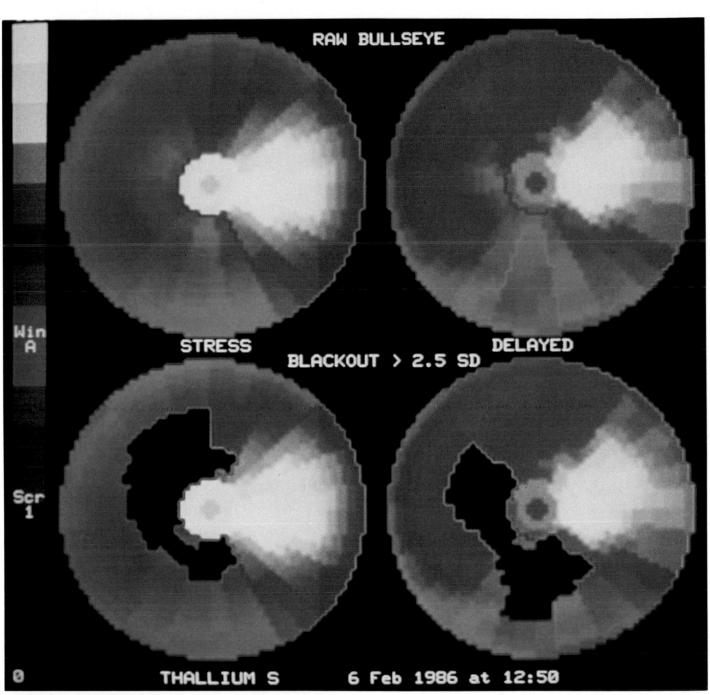

A bull's-eye analysis of a diseased heart has been developed at Emory University School of Medicine to detect abnormalities and myocardial infarction. The colors indicate the amount of thallium uptake and deviation from the norm. The two left images were obtained under stress; the two right images were obtained 3 hours later at rest. Blackout areas indicate decreased blood supply to the heart muscle. This is a SPECT-thallium study.

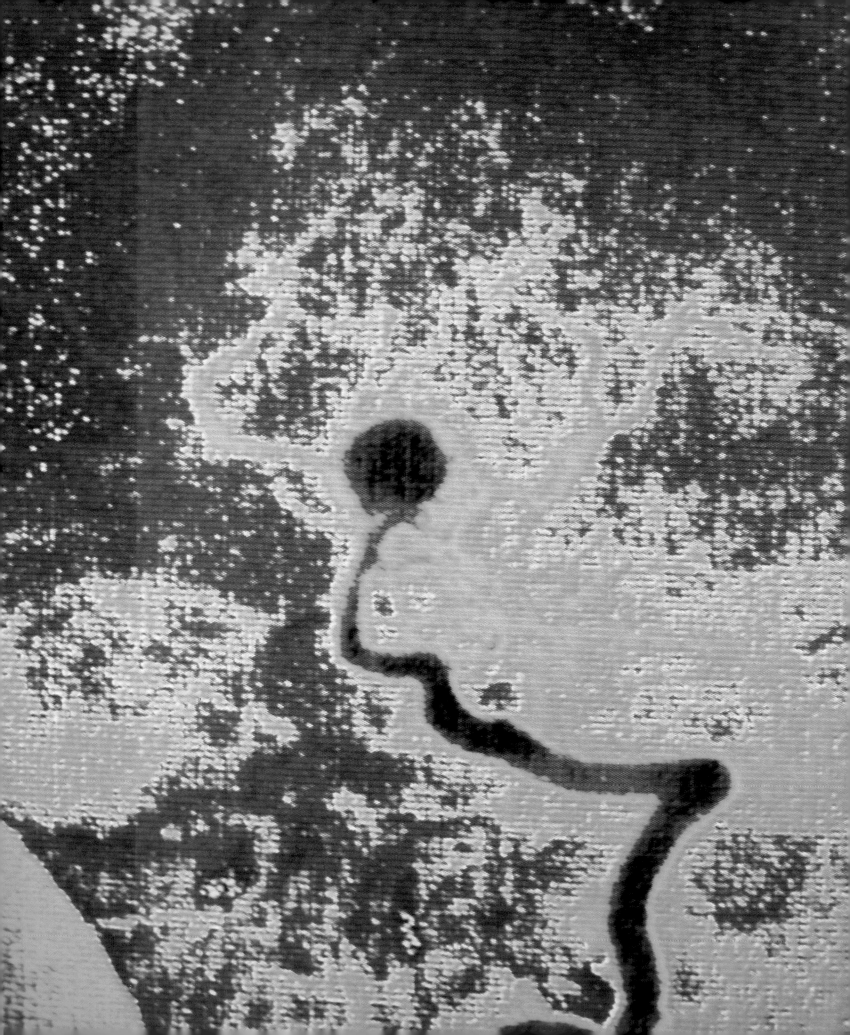

V. INTERVENTIONAL RADIOLOGY

"Surgery without a knife"

O
ne of the newest and most promising areas of medical imaging is the field of interventional radiology. It offers the patient an alternative to surgery and the long healing process that surgery usually entails.

Viewing the human circulatory system as interconnected roadways or a vast river complex with countless tributaries, the radiologist has devised methods of entering and traveling within the system to reach almost every internal recess of the body. The utilization of these arterial passageways is at the heart of interventional radiology.

But before wide application of this technique became possible, a method of seeing inside the body's roadways had to be developed. Angiography, an imaging technique that produces clear views of flowing blood or its blockage by narrowed vessels, gives radiologists that inner vision essential for interventional procedures. Angiography involves the injection into the vessels of a contrast agent containing iodine that is opaque to x rays; the shadow this creates allows doctors to see the flow of blood.

Recently, angiographic images have been enhanced by computer manipulation (digital subtraction angiography or DSA). Before injection of the contrast agent, an x-ray image is obtained and stored in a computer. After injection, a second image is obtained highlighting the flowing blood as revealed by the contrast agent. The computer then superimposes the two images exactly and subtracts image one from image two, leaving only a sharp

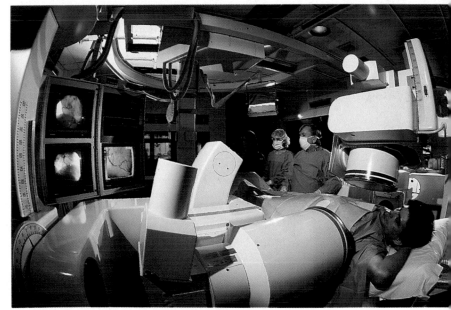

A two-for-one scanner, the digital biplane angioscope at East Jefferson General Hospital in New Orleans provides views of the heart from two different angles. A screen can present four images: two live views of the heart, one digital recorded picture, and a display — here dark — of physiological data.

An artery at the base of the brain balloons with a dangerous aneurysm (left) in an image enhanced by digital subtraction angiography (DSA).

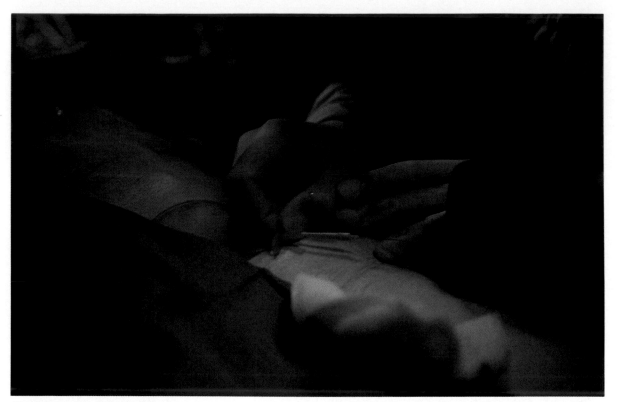

The hands of Dr. Alex Berenstein at NYU Medical Center deftly thread a catheter into a patient who has a huge pelvic growth. He cut the blood supply to the growth by sealing off the supply with a glue not unlike ``crazy glue.'' DSA permits him to see exactly what is happening within the veins and arteries.

picture of blood vessels such as the coronary arteries, the main suppliers of blood to the heart.

A common surgical procedure in the United States today is coronary bypass surgery. In this procedure, blood vessels that are clogged with fatty or calcified material are bypassed using other vessels surgically removed from another part of the body, usually the leg. In recent years more than 200,000 operations of this kind have been performed annually at an average cost of about $25,000, for a staggering national price tag totaling some $5 billion.

With the help of angiography and a procedure called angioplasty, many of these operations can now be avoided.

In coronary artery angioplasty, a catheter is threaded through a blood vessel in the arm or groin. Using the fluoroscopic images on a TV screen, the catheter is guided into a coronary artery. At this time, the contrast agent is injected providing a clear image of the arterial blockage. A second, smaller catheter inserted through the first carries a tiny balloon to the spot. The outer catheter is pulled back and the balloon is inflated until it compresses the materials clogging the artery and again allows the blood to supply the heart muscle.

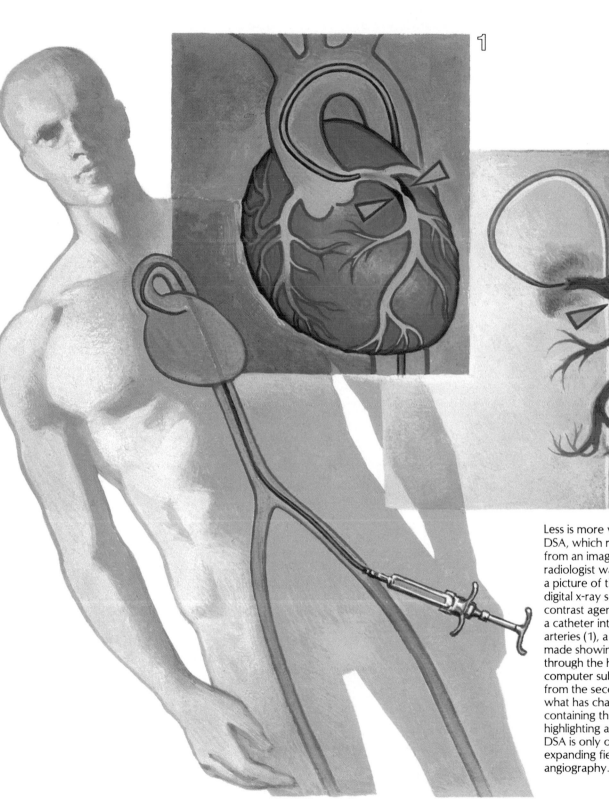

Less is more with the wizardry of DSA, which removes everything from an image except what the radiologist wants to examine. First a picture of the heart is made by a digital x-ray scanner. Next, as a contrast agent is injected through a catheter into the coronary arteries (1), a second x-ray image is made showing the agent flowing through the heart's vessels. A computer subtracts the first image from the second, leaving only what has changed — blood vessels containing the agent (2) — and highlighting a blockage (arrows). DSA is only one application of the expanding field of computed angiography.

Made by digital subtraction angiography, a color-enhanced close-up picture of Dr. James Quinn's left coronary artery shows one branch, at far left, to be totally blocked. A blood clot stopped the flow of blood when it lodged against a deposit of plaque. Enlarged by exercise, his other arteries enabled him to survive the heart attack.

To remove the clot, a catheter was threaded into the heart through a blood vessel in the groin — while watching its progress on a digital angiography unit — and a dissolving agent was injected at the point of blockage. To open the artery further, a second catheter, fitted with a small balloon, was inserted through the first. Gently inflating the balloon, the plaque is compressed against the wall of the artery, slightly stretching its lining. A follow-up image shows the branch completely open again.

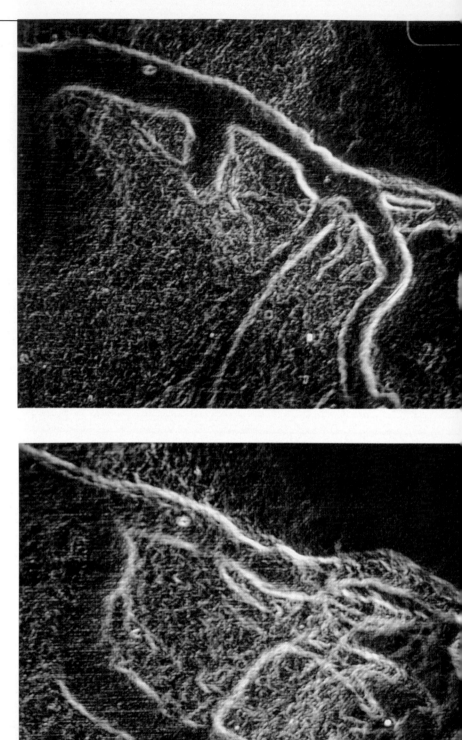

To learn about one patient's experience with angioplasty, I contacted James Quinn, a 65-year-old professor at Louisiana State University School of Dentistry. Dr. Quinn did everything right: he ran three miles a day, watched his cholesterol, and was a nonsmoker and nondrinker of normal weight. His last treadmill stress test, in 1983, was normal, as was a nuclear heart scan the same year.

At 2 AM on January 9, 1986, he awoke to deep chest pains and arm numbness. At 2:30 AM his wife Judy called an ambulance that rushed him to the clinic. He was given emergency treatment, and by 9:30 AM the balloon catheter was inserted and dilated. Immediately, it relieved a 100% blockage of the blood supply to a branch of the left coronary artery.

A week later Dr. Quinn repeated a treadmill test without chest pain. He has suffered no further heart damage and has been skiing, plays tennis regularly, and again runs three miles a day. The quality of his life has been restored, and now—almost three years post-angioplasty—he is still in the best of health.

Laser angioplasty

Although coronary angioplasty has helped thousands and in many cases made bypass surgery unnecessary, there are two major drawbacks that should be mentioned. One is "snowplowing" where the material clogging the artery is simply pushed ahead of the penetrating catheter only to remain a continuing problem; a second complication is the possibility of damaging the wall of an artery, with the catheter itself causing hemorrhage.

Another of the newest techniques in interventional medicine, laser angioplasty, may at least be a partial solution to the "snowplowing" problem. Since the laser vaporizes the undesired material, the threat of the particles causing problems elsewhere can be reduced. Various types of laser catheters for this procedure are being studied. In many cases, the laser is used to heat the tip of a catheter to a temperature great enough to melt a passage through the obstructing plaque. This passage can later become a channel through which successful balloon angioplasty procedures can be performed.

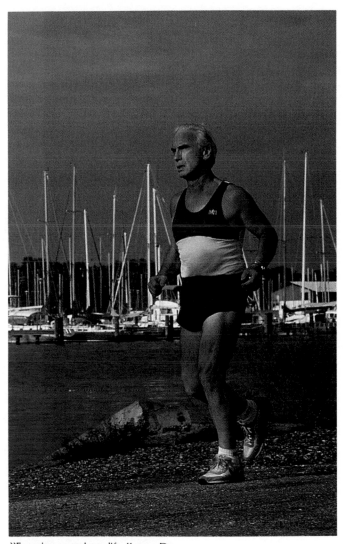

"Exercise saved my life," says Dr. James Quinn of New Orleans who, for several days in 1986, felt a tightness in his chest during his daily three-mile run. "Then zap, one night I had this pain," he says. It was a major heart attack.

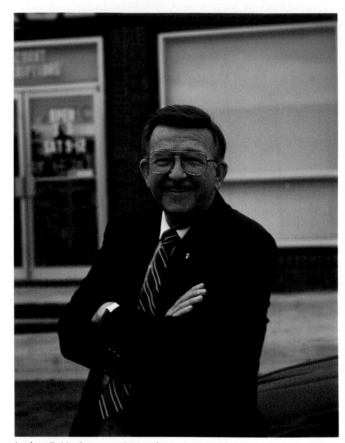

Luther E. Hodge, a registered pharmacist and practicing minister in Clarksville, Arkansas suffered severe leg pains shortly after his bypass surgery for nine coronary blockages. Angiography revealed occlusion of the main arteries in both legs. A laser was used to restore circulation on two separate operations. "I went back to work the next day," he happily reported.

One area of easy application for the laser is in the arterial system supplying the legs. Since the major artery in the lower leg (popliteal) is quite large and linear (without curves and turns), straight access to an obstruction is possible.

To get a patient's view on laser therapy, I traveled to Clarksville, Arkansas, west of Little Rock, to talk to Luther E. Hodge, a registered pharmacist and practicing minister in the Church of Christ.

Luther's problems started in 1980 with severe chest pains and frequent faintness and loss of breath. He delayed medical attention, but finally (1985) took a stress test followed the next day by an arteriogram that clearly displayed nine coronary blockages. On November 17, 1985, six bypass grafts were implanted in Luther's heart. He felt better, but a month later was troubled by leg pain which got so severe that he could not walk at all. A friend told him about the experimental laser work being done at the University of Arkansas Medical School in Little Rock where he was referred to Dr. Ernest Ferris, Chief of Radiology, and to Dr. Tim McCowan, Resident and an RSNA Research Fellow.

On April 23, 1987, laser angioplasty was performed in Little Rock. Angiography had discovered major blockages in both legs. The left leg was approached first, and a 1-cm incision was made in the groin. A needle opened the femoral artery and the catheter containing the metal-tipped laser, carried in a 2-mm fiberoptic bundle, was inserted (a protective sheath is inserted into the artery for the first 15 cm). Luther's popliteal artery, which was about 7 mm in diameter, was blocked about 40 cm from the entry point. Luther told me he remained fully conscious throughout the procedure and was only given morphine for back pain that had been chronic even before the operation.

During the 4½-hour procedure, an argon laser with a metal tip was brought to a temperature of 400°C to literally melt away the obstruction in the main artery (tissue vaporizes at 1,000°C). Bursts of heat of 10-second duration were given after which progress was evaluated by angiography. Almost a 4″ segment of the artery was opened. After the laser made an initial opening, a balloon was inserted to

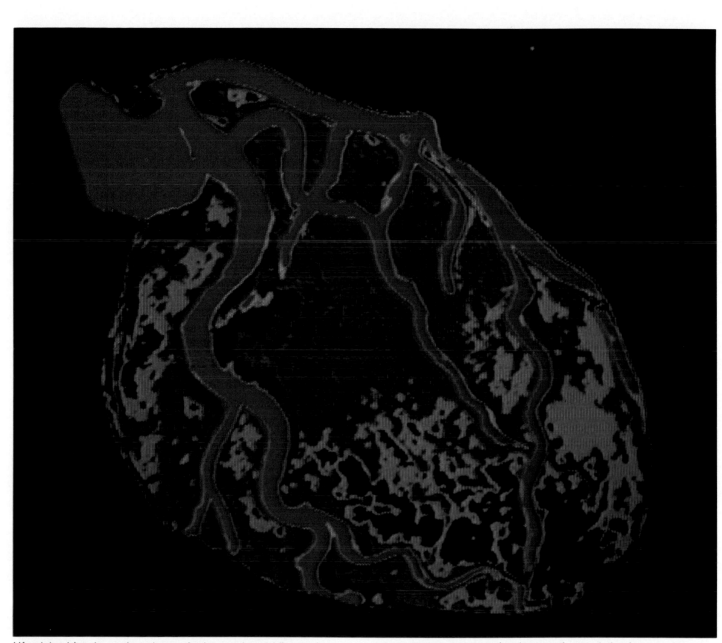

Life-giving blood vessels embrace the heart of a middle-aged man in this picture made by digital subtraction angiography (DSA). Filled with a substance opaque to x rays, the left coronary artery — bright red in this color-enhanced view — feeds a network of smaller vessels deep in the walls of the heart muscle. The red pool at left is the aortic root. A constriction in the coronary artery at top, appearing as a break, has choked off 60% of the blood supply to the lower part of the heart.

A computer measures the degree of constriction by converting the image into digital code and comparing it with others made from different angles. It also measures the rate at which blood diffuses into the heart muscle, giving doctors a good indication of whether or not a heart attack is likely to occur.

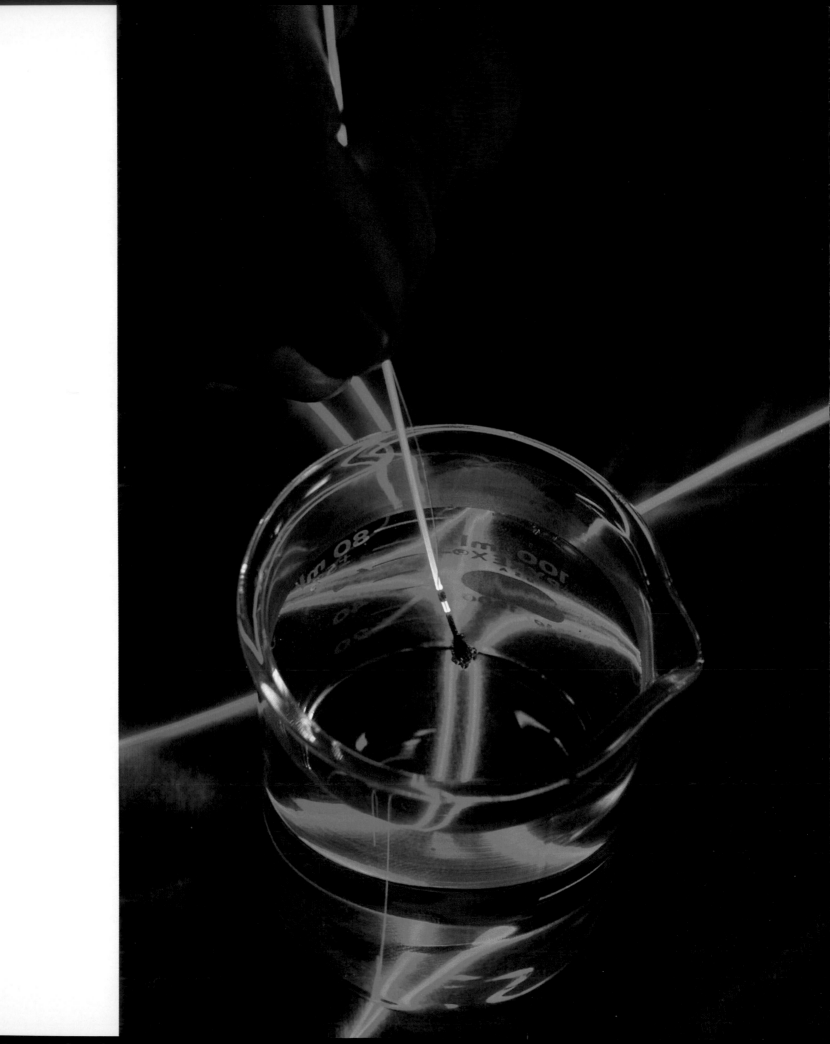

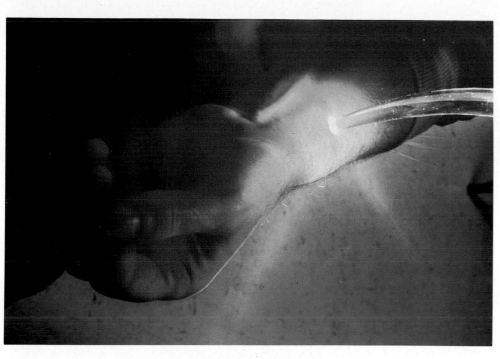

Laser energy is carried in either glass or a fiber optic filament to be used in treatment of skin cancer (above) or to be inserted into a catheter (below) for internal use. Top photo shows removal of wart from arm of Dr. Leon Goldman, a pioneer in medical laser applications at Cincinnati Children's Hospital, University of Cincinnati.

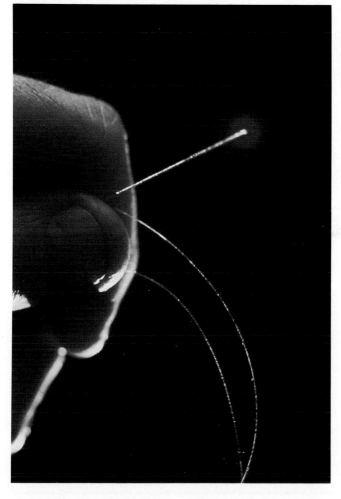

An argon laser (far left) with a "hot tip" which heats to a temperature of 400°C is used to melt the plaque found in blocked arteries. The laser (which is pulsed during the operation) is pretested in a beaker of water.

make an even larger passage for the blood supply to the lower leg.

Just three months later, on July 23, 1987, the right leg received the laser treatment. In this case only a 2" segment of the popliteal artery was occluded and the operation lasted only 1½ hours.

"I went to work the day after the procedure," he told me. Hodge is a strong advocate of laser medicine. And although he sold his chain of five pharmacies, at 62 he divides his time between a pharmacy management consulting business and his work for his church.

Dr. Mark Wholey, a radiologist at Shadyside Hospital near Pittsburgh, told me of another interventional tool under investigation. It is a tiny

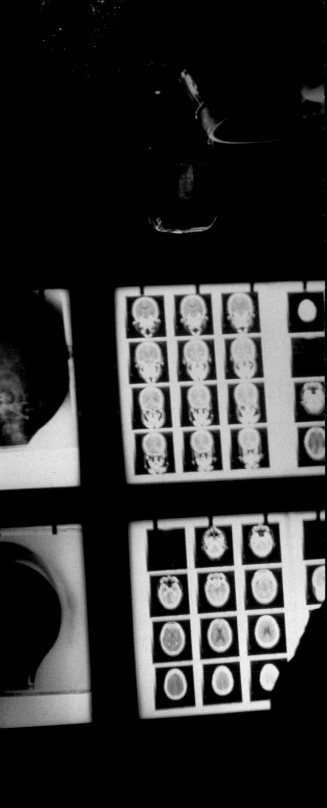

"roto rooter" drilling wire, only 3 mm in diameter, that functions like a high-speed drill. Operating at 150,000 rpm, it is a catheter with a cutting tip that can open occlusions as long as 40 cm (16"). A newer wire (athrolytic reperfusion wire) that both cuts and opens is as tiny as 0.9 mm and revolves at 80,000 rpm.

Eminent interventionalist Dr. Bob White, formerly of Johns Hopkins University Medical School and now Chairman of the Department of Radiology at Yale University Medical School, told me about several other applications of interventional radiology such as drainage or removal of abscess, blood, or liquid, and the infusion of drugs to dissolve clots, treat cancers, or stop bleeding. "We radiologists are wonderful picture getters," he told me, "now we must use this imaging ability to treat."

More than anyone else, Dr. Charles T. Dotter (1920–1985) deserves a salute as the founder and chief stimulator of interventional radiology. His creative mind, exploring spirit, untiring energy, and technical skill led radiologists into new territories. To underscore the rapidity of this progress, Dr. White told me of his first visit to Europe to meet another pioneer in balloon angioplasty, Dr. A. R. Gruentzig of Zurich. "In his dark, dingy basement I found two guys handcrafting the balloons which were the world's total supply of balloons for coronary angioplasty. That was just 10 years ago. It was a great loss to radiologic science when Dr. Gruentzig was killed in an airplane crash in 1985."

Guided by pictures of the brain unimaginable 20 years ago, Dr. Paul O'Boynick (second from right) at the University of Kansas Medical Center delicately implants a tube in a patient's skull to drain excess fluid. Dr. Dwane Beckenhauer (left) prepares an incision where the tube, after being threaded beneath the skin, will be inserted into the abdominal cavity for the fluid to be continuously absorbed. Behind them are images of another patient (CT, MRI, and conventional angiography) illustrating the variety of information available to neurosurgeons in modern operating rooms.

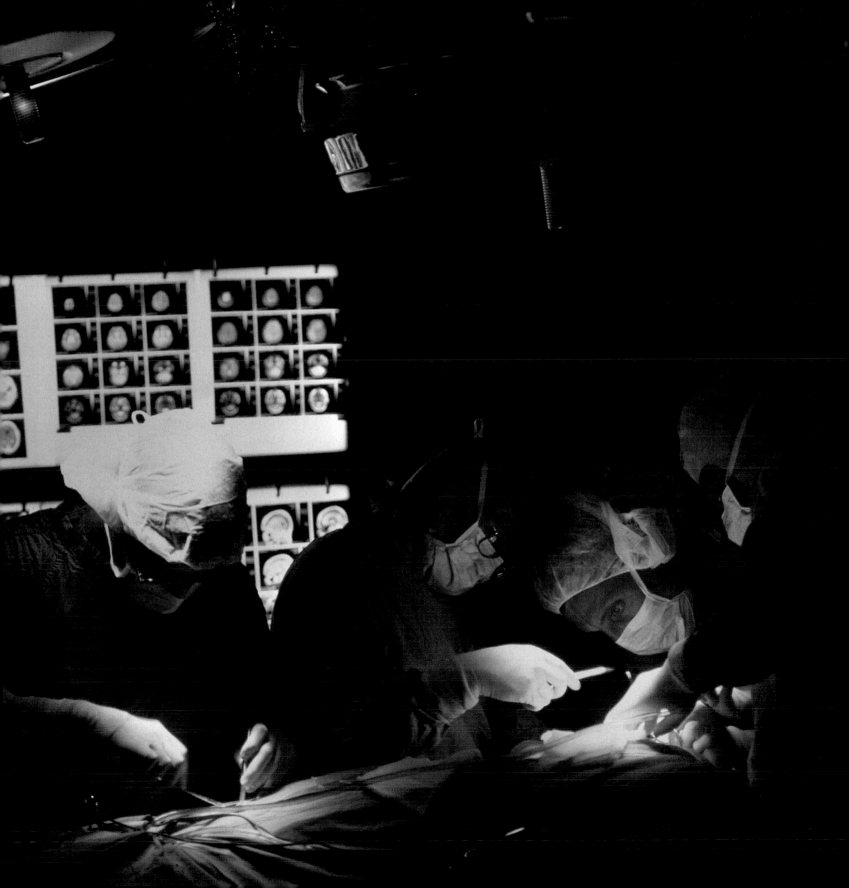

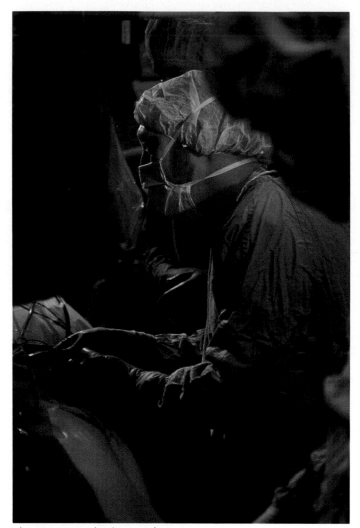

A master at navigating a catheter inside the body, Dr. Alex Berenstein, professor of Radiology and Director of Surgical Neuroangiography at NYU Medical Center and Bellevue Hospital, has pioneered a technique of depositing a 95% ethanol solution directly onto venous lesions to shrink and destroy them.

Just as angiography helps in procedures to open up arteries, there are times when it is used in techniques for closing off blood supply to abnormal tissues or organs.

A leading practitioner of this application is Dr. Alex Berenstein, at NYU Medical Center in New York City. While serving his surgical internship in Israel in 1970, he became fascinated with the practice of drip irrigation used by Israeli farmers to conserve water in the desert. "Why can't this drop-by-drop method be applied in surgery?" he thought.

One day he applied a small amount of Gelfoam—a sealing gelatin sponge—to stop the bleeding in a patient's stomach. Guided by DSA equipment, he now uses catheters, some of his own design, to inject tiny drops of isobutyl-2-cyanoacrylate (a strong adhesive) to seal off the blood supply to growing tumors or ruptured vessels. He also uses the technique in delicate cases of brain hemorrhage.

I spent a day with Dr. Berenstein in his crowded operating room in New York and came away with the conviction that in his profession very few people have the talent to do what he is doing.

He schedules two operations a day—roughly 400 a year. His patients come to him from all over the world; the greatest number of them requiring the sealing-off or embolizing technique that he has perfected. Besides the isobutyl, he also uses tiny balloons as sealants and shunts to divert blood supply.

The first patient of the day was a pretty, 24-year-old woman who had a huge mass just outside the uterus in the pelvic area. Because of the tumor's location, surgery had been ruled out since it could render her unable to have children.

Interventional treatment of the fetus before birth has been applied to such life-threatening conditions as *hydrocephalus* (fluid buildup in the brain) and *hydronephrosis* (a blockage of the urinary tract).

This computer-enhanced image illustrates injection that passes through abdomen, uterus, and into fetal bladder.

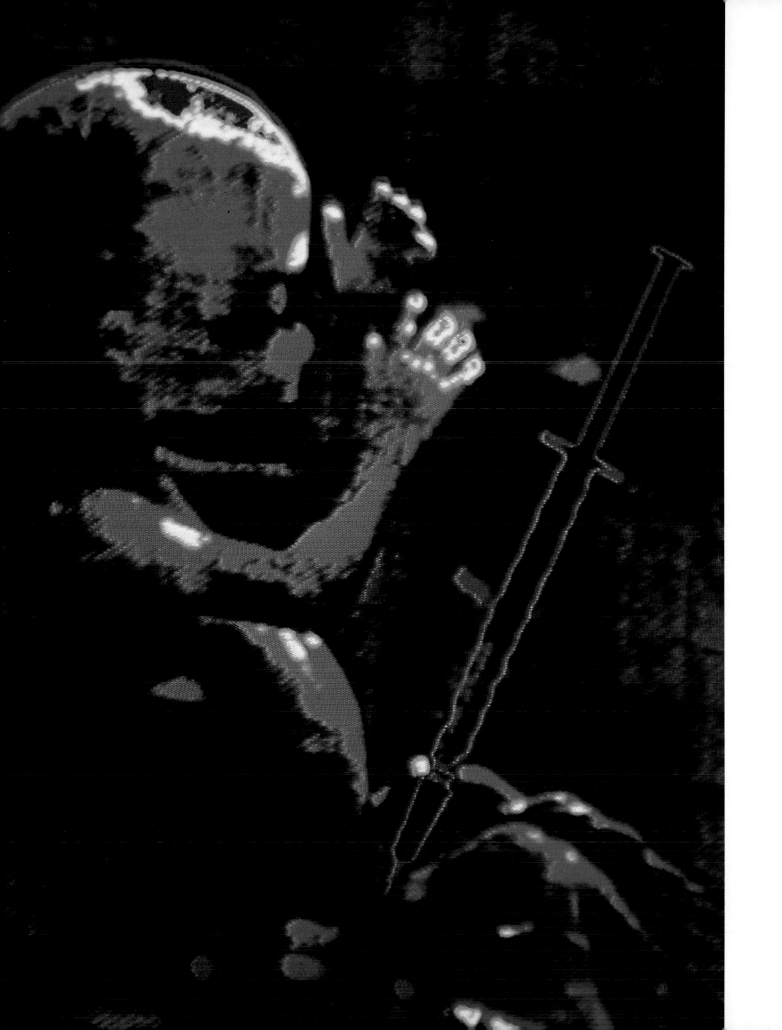

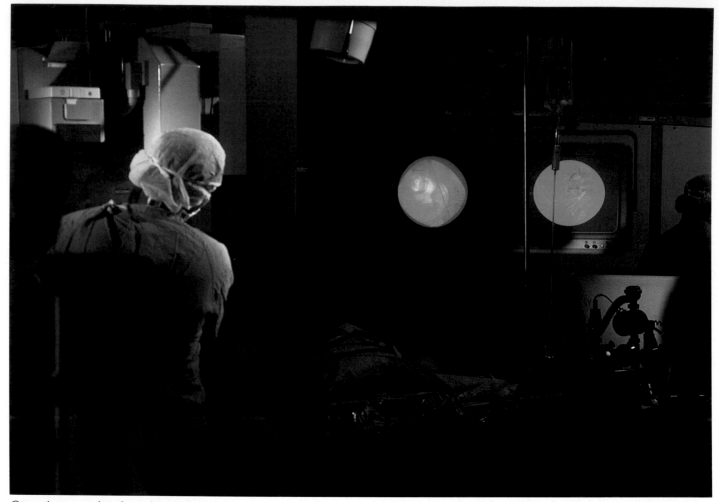

Operating procedure for pelvic mass at
Catheter Lab of NYU Medical Center. Dr.
Berenstein (left) feels "we are at the beginning
of a whole new era in interventional medicine."
Monitors (rear) give two views of arteries in the
pelvis — one computer processed image, one
conventional image. Dr. Berenstein does two
operations daily, about 400 a year.

The patient was sedated. In a tense, five-hour
operation, Dr. Berenstein carefully threaded his
catheters through the veins and arteries of the body
to the huge cluster of tangled vessels that were
supplying the tumor with blood and allowing it to
grow.

"Cut off the blood supply to this tumor and it
will fade away," Dr. Berenstein told me.

While watching his DSA monitor and
periodically injecting small amounts of contrast
material, he used the catheters, some only 2 mm in
diameter, to deposit the sealant in five different
locations. A total of 3.8 cc of isobutyl was used; its

amount carefully monitored and precisely dispensed
since it sets rock-hard in just two to eight seconds.
Too much glue would be toxic to kidneys; too little
would allow continued blood supply to the tumor.

Almost immediately I could see the results of
the procedure. Blood at five strategic points had
stopped flowing to the mass. It would die from
starvation.

In his more recent work, Dr. Berenstein has
been experimenting with the use of alcohol by direct
injection through catheters to destroy malignant
tumors. If successful over a long period of evaluation,
this method could be another life saver for patients
with tumors that are otherwise inoperable.

"We are only at the very beginning," claims
Berenstein. "Most every day we are doing
something that has never been done before."

Another application of interventional radiology
is practiced by Dr. Fred Stitik, Professor and
Chairman of Radiology, East Virginia Medical School,

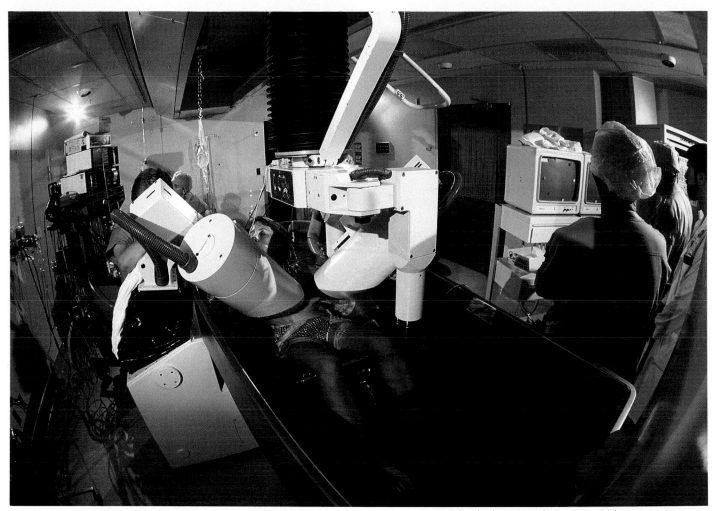

A "depth charge explosion" crumbles stones into sand. Lithotripsy for removal of kidney stones is performed at the University of Arizona Medical Center by Dr. George Drock and six attendants. Under full anesthetic the patient is immersed into a 50-gallon water bath. A shock wave is pulsed into the area of the stone and slowly disintegrates it. The physician applies from 700–2,000 shock exposures. Recovery is very fast; patients usually require only two to three days of hospitalization.

Norfolk, Virginia. He is one of the experts in needle aspiration.

Using biplane fluoroscopy (two x-ray units at 90° to one another), he carefully guides a hollow needle, 1 or 2 mm in diameter and about 20 cm in length, to the area of an undetermined mass. Suction is applied and a small sample of the mass is removed. A pathologist present in the radiology room then does an immediate microscopic evaluation of the mass to determine whether it is benign or malignant. Taking only 45 minutes to an hour to complete, a needle aspiration procedure is most often done on an outpatient basis thus avoiding the trauma and cost of surgery.

Another new tool, extracorporeal shock wave lithotripsy, is used by the radiologist/urologist team to treat patients with kidney stones and eliminates the need for surgery in a growing number of patients. Initially developed in Europe, it uses an electrically generated shock wave to literally pulverize kidney stones. These stones usually lodge in the kidneys or block the ureter that drains the kidneys' fluids (urine) into the bladder.

Anyone who has suffered from kidney stones knows the extreme pain that accompanies this disorder. Surgery is often difficult. Now, when possible, lithotripsy has become the treatment of choice for over 100,000 patients in the United States annually. At this writing, over 500,000 patients have been treated worldwide since 1984. The installation and equipment are expensive and require up to a $2.5-million investment by the hospital.

In operation, the equipment consists of two x-ray tubes for viewing the stones before and after they disintegrate, and an electrode operating at about 20 kilovolts that produces a spark. The patient is immersed in a water-filled, stainless steel tub. The shock wave from the pulsed spark is transferred through the water into the patient. The wave, synchronized to the patient's heartbeat (the R-wave), disintegrates the kidney stone(s). One patient described the aftereffects to me: "When I awoke I felt like I had been hit in the back with a baseball bat." But the soreness hardly compares with that suffered previously from kidney stone surgery.

Dr. Howard Pollack at the University of Pennsylvania Hospital in Philadelphia has a nationwide reputation in this field. He told me that the procedure works on most stone removals with the following exceptions: 1), when a patient is too large for the tub; 2), when the location of the stone is such that the spark generator (focused hydraulic electromechanical energy) cannot focus on the stone; or 3), when the location of the kidney in an obese person (over 300 lbs) rules out its application.

Kidney stones vary in size. Dr. Pollack showed me one, a "stag horn," that filled the entire collecting system of a kidney. Rough and jagged with sharp, tentacle-like fingers, it was about 3" in diameter. It required three sessions of lithotripsy during a period of one week to remove it entirely (the number of wave bursts is limited; an excessive number can cause kidney damage).

As many as five stone removals a day are performed in Dr. Pollack's department on one machine. About 15% of patients tend to reform stones after a year or more and then return for another treatment.

In a new development in Philadelphia, Dr. Peter Malet is awaiting the installation of equipment that will distintegrate gallstones in the gallbladder just as kidney stones are now removed. The equipment will base its imaging component on ultrasound, since gallstones are of a different chemical consistency than kidney stones and are not visible to the x-ray viewing systems of the lithotripsy units now in use. The new machine will not require a water bath, but will use the same spark-gap discharge, "the

antisubmarine depth charge explosive technique" as Dr. Malet describes it.

I witnessed a stone removal procedure at the University of Arizona Medical Center in Tucson. The patient was Carol Cameron, a 27-year-old administrative assistant to a neurologist in Albuquerque, New Mexico. Carol had a history of kidney stones. She had one previous lithotripsy treatment, two nephrostomies (a surgical entry through the back of the patient to remove the stone), and one basket removal procedure. At another time, one stone passed through the bladder normally without intervention. She described herself as hypercalcemic, wherein the body naturally absorbs too much calcium (for reasons that remain unknown).

I saw Carol at about 7:30 AM in the modern, multi-million dollar installation that had opened in May 1986. She would be the 506th patient to use the facility. Two million dollars had been spent to electrically shield and soundproof the room which was about 30' × 40' in dimension. Seven doctors were in attendance (four were trainee observers). The key players were Dr. George Drock, Chief of Urology; Stephen Alder, a radiologic technician; and Dr. Steve Cardon, the anesthesiologist.

Shortly after I got Carol's permission to photograph the procedure, she was given a full anesthetic. A 10" stent or flexible plastic tube was then passed into her bladder and up the left ureter to her kidney. The purpose of the stent was to widen the ureter and to permit the easy passage of stone fragments out of the kidney. While seated in a hydraulic reclining chair, she was slowly lowered into the huge, stainless steel, water-filled bath tub. At the bottom of the tub were the electronic shock wave generator and two x-ray generator tubes covered with white balloon protectors.

The first instruction to the team came from the radiologic technician who instructed the nurse to "balloons up." The balloons were inflated to provide a watertight covering for the x-ray generators. Carol was positioned so that her kidney was directly above the generator with only her head remaining above water. Over the tub were two huge gantry arms that contained image intensifiers to display the x-ray

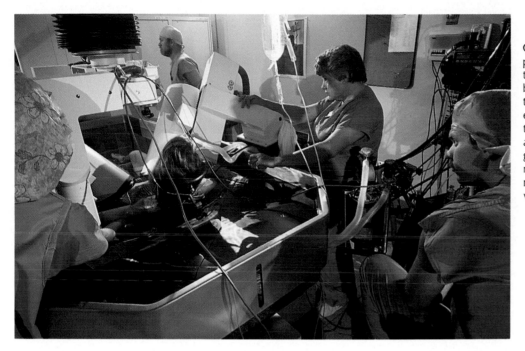

Carol Cameron, this pretty blond patient, has now had three lithotripsy treatments. Latest equipment now being installed replaces the water tank with a water belt. Other equipment has been developed to treat gallstones. This latest device uses an ultrasound viewing system since gallstones, unlike kidney stones, are not visible by x-ray. One hundred million people suffer from gallstones worldwide.

image. The success of the operation could be easily viewed on a TV monitor during the entire procedure. It revealed the slow destruction of the ¼" stone.

The treatment took about a half hour. During that time about 2,000 shock waves timed to synchronize with the heart's action (about one a second) were given. Each time the shock wave was turned on a blue flash illuminated the water in the tub. At 10:00 AM the procedure ended and Carol was taken to the recovery room.

About 5:00 PM that same day I dropped by to see her in her hospital room. She said she felt fine. She did have a little nausea from the anesthetic and a soreness in her back in the area of her kidney. The spot on her back closest to the kidney was black-and-blue. She was released from the hospital two days later.

Many patients make repeated trips to hospitals for stone removal, some as often as one a year. To date, no conclusive data have been collected on prolonged or repeated use of lithotripsy or possible kidney damage that can result.

As previously mentioned, Carol had stones removed by a nephrostomy technique on two previous occasions. In this technique, a needle is inserted into the back and penetrates the kidney. The needle is hollow and carries a viewing lens, a shock wave generator that pulverizes the stone, and a suction device that removes the stone debris after it is pulverized. Of the two procedures, lithotripsy is preferred since less kidney damage results from the shock wave than from needle penetration.

In the future, new equipment now being developed in Germany will use a "water cushion" instead of the "bath tub" immersion technique. And when FDA approval for this technique is received, a general anesthetic will no longer be required. Since 1987 all lithotripsy procedures in Europe have been performed without an anesthetic.

The rule of thumb in medicine has always been that new developments work on a 30-year cycle—the time it takes to invent, research, test, and finally approve and apply a new technology. In interventional radiology this timetable is being drastically altered; afterall, as few as 15 years ago most of the interventional techniques mentioned herein did not even exist. As one interventional radiologist told me, "we are no longer a few loonies out on the fringe. We are finally being accepted by the medical community."

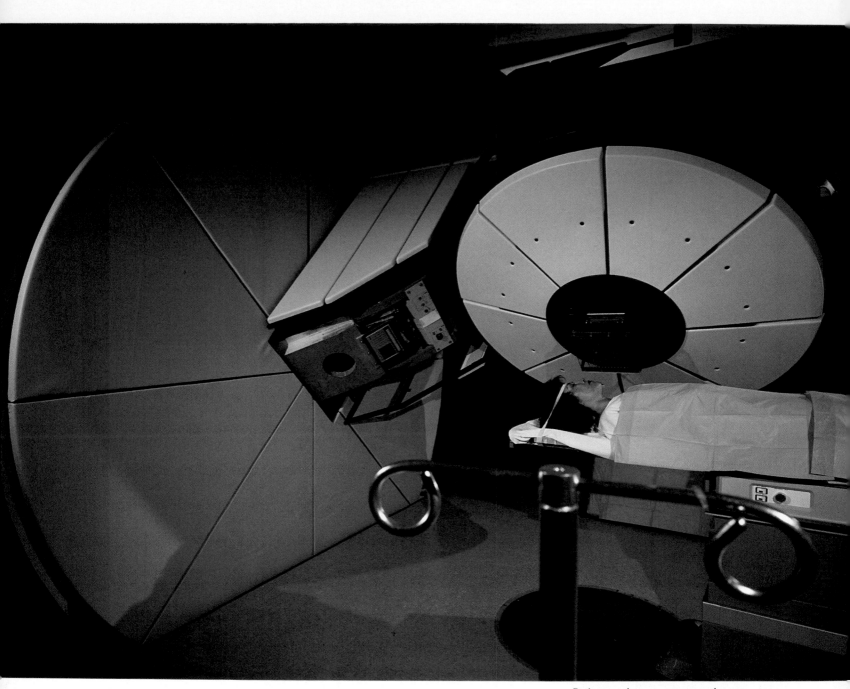

Patient undergoes neutron therapy at new experimental facility at the University of California Center for Health Sciences in Los Angeles. Short bursts of radiation are used to kill cancer. Newest energy sources in treatment are neutrons, protons, and heavy ions that bombard and kill cancers.

VI. RADIATION THERAPY

"Radiation cures cancer"

Radiation therapy (also called therapeutic radiology) employs many forms of ionizing radiations to kill cancer cells. Either alone or in conjunction with surgery and/or chemotherapy, it will be used to treat more than half of the 1 million cancer patients in the United States next year.

The technologies and techniques of radiation therapy are many. Widely used is a huge linear accelerator with a generator head, set on a revolving gantry, that directs electron and photon rays to targeted cancer tissue. The patient lies perfectly still in a precise position so that the radiation can be accurately delivered. Because some damage occurs to surrounding healthy tissue (the beam often must pass through healthy tissue to get to the cancerous tissue), the beam usually approaches the tumor from several directions. Using this method, the focused beam delivers a 100% dose to the cancer and a much smaller dose to the surrounding tissue. Radiation kills cells by the ionization of molecules that results in physical and chemical change in the targeted tissue. Biological effects are directly related to the amount of absorbed energy. Therapy is usually administered for a few minutes daily over a period of several weeks. The total dose in the diseased area can sometimes reach or exceed 60 Gy (an absorbed dose of radiation).

In addition to high-energy, focused beams (cobalt machine or linear accelerator), there are other methods of delivering radiation. In brachytherapy, radium, or radioactive cesium, iridium, or other

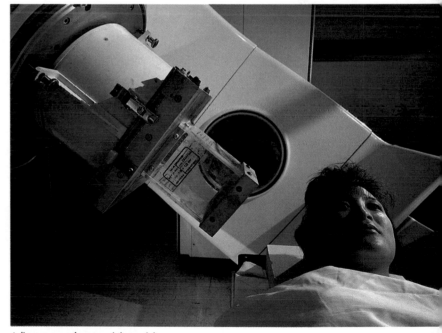

A linear accelerator (above) is a modern, standard treatment device for radiation therapy. Precise delivery of radiation for short periods of time saves the lives of an estimated 250,000 cancer patients yearly. An aperature head (left) limits radiation to a specific area.

implants are put in direct contact with or inserted into a tumor for a period of treatment that can last as long as a few days. Its use is limited to specific places in the body (the uterus, vagina, rectum or prostate, for example) where either surgery or an orifice permit insertion of the materials. Some of these implants, consisting of radioactive iodine or gold, are left in place permanently.

Another method of radiation treatment is the use of isotopes that have a fairly short half-life. Most commonly used are liquid forms of phosphorous 32 and iodine 131 which can be introduced into various body cavities (the peritoneal cavity containing the intestines or the pleural cavity around the lungs).

Because cancer affects so many of our lives and radiation therapy's role in the treatment of cancer is so substantial, I wanted to find out about the latest developments and approaches in this vital specialty.

Dr. Zvi Fuks is Chairman of Radiation Oncology at Memorial Sloan-Kettering Cancer Center in New York City. One of the largest radiation treatment centers in the United States, it handles 3,000 new patients each year. The center has been part of a multi-institutional investigative effort contracted by the National Cancer Institute to develop precise 3-D radiotherapy planning and treatment by delivering photon beams that accurately conform to the shape of the tumor target.

Megavoltage radiation therapy, which includes cobalt units and linear accelerators operating at 4 to 50 million volts, has been used since about 1950 to deliver high-energy beams of photons and electrons that penetrate the body and destroy cancerous tumors.

The current conventional techniques of 2-D radiation therapy employ multiple radiation fields aimed at the tumor from various angles but in a single plane of the body.

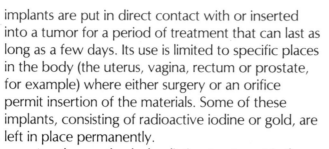

A laser beam indicates the exact position of delivery of either electron or photon rays to a cancer victim. Since prolonged exposure can kill healthy tissue, extreme care is taken to achieve minimum exposure to healthy tissues and a killing exposure to cancer tissues.

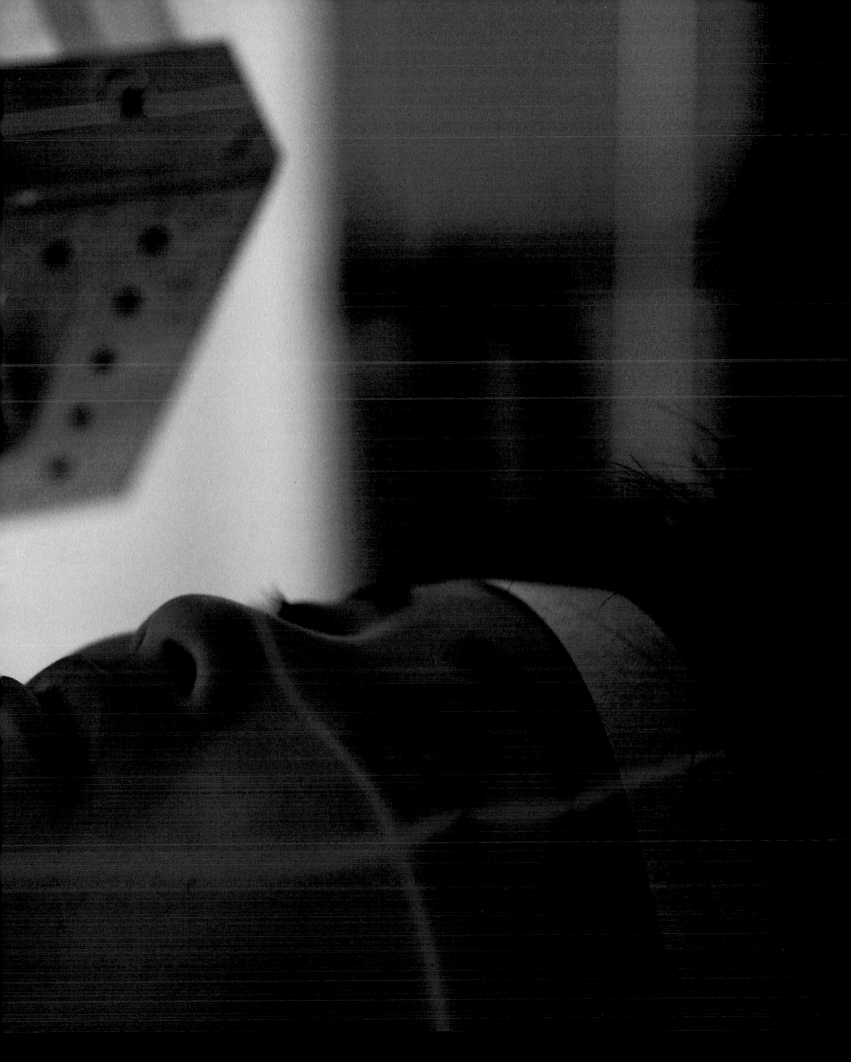

The process starts with the aid of a specialized diagnostic machine called a simulator. Using this method, the adequacy of the planned treatment is carefully assessed and modifications can be made to obtain the best treatment possible under the circumstances. But due to the limitations of conventional diagnostic x-ray methods "our confidence in the true dimension and location of the tumor was not absolute," Dr. Fuks remarked. Therefore, in conventional 2-D treatment a large safety margin around the tumor has to be included in the treatment field. Obviously, this generous margin included areas of sensitive normal tissue. In the process, normal tissues suffered significant damage; thus, normal tissue tolerance has always been the limiting factor in the application of successful treatment. As an example, the lung, liver, and heart are sufficiently sensitive to the effects of radiation that the capacity to treat tumors adjacent to them is limited.

"Because of the limitations of conventional 2-D methods, potentially curable tumors sometimes recur," Dr. Fuks explained. Of an estimated 220,000 patients in 1988 who could be radiation curable, only half will in fact be cured. Of the remaining patients (110,000), it is estimated that 67,000 will not be cured because the radiation treatment missed part of the tumor.

But with the advent of CT, the accuracy of treatment will improve. "We can now define more precisely the true extent and position of the tumor by obtaining a series of CT scans throughout the tumor region" explained Dr. Radhe Mohan, a medical physicist who has worked with Dr. Fuks to develop the system. "With the aid of specialized computer programs, we can precisely reconstruct the 3-D configuration of the tumor, look at it from any side and geometry, define its borders, and determine its relationship to other organs. This will enable us to aim radiation fields from a number of directions, with the shape of each radiation field chosen to best conform to the tumor and avoid damage of normal tissue."

"We are sharpening the x-ray knife to remove the tumor. We don't know how much of an improvement over our current failure rate is achievable. It will take a few years to tell," explained Dr. Fuks.

The planning of 3-D treatment uses new techniques such as the "Beam's Eye View." It is as if the human eye was placed at the exact position of the origin of the radiation and watched where it went.

Another new development that will assist in continuously shaping the radiation field as the beam moves around the tumor is the multi-leafed collimator. It has a series of ½" metal strips that function like the diaphragm of a camera lens, producing an aperture that resembles the exact shape of a tumor. This baffle system is placed between the x-ray source and the patient. "Up to 80 leaves guided by motors can duplicate any tumor in size and shape," Dr. Fuks further explained.

Now actual patient treatment using 3-D conformal radiotherapy has begun at Memorial Sloan-Kettering Cancer Center and at other centers throughout the United States: the University of Michigan Medical Center in Ann Arbor, the University of Pennsylvania Medical School in Philadelphia, the University of North Carolina Medical Center in Chapel Hill, the Mallinckrodt Institute in St. Louis, the Massachusetts General Hospital in Boston, and the University of Washington in Seattle.

Many problems remain to be solved; among them, developing better, more efficient computer software, optimizing the design of the fields, improving the control of the machines, and accurately assessing the results of the new radiation treatment.

For the future, Dr. Fuks sees even further improvement in imaging techniques for 3-D planning and therapy; CT, MR, ultrasound, radionuclide imaging such as PET, or monoclonal antibody imaging. All might be used independently or in combination to image the exact area to be treated.

The "treatment plan" is central to radiation therapy. Each day, a department team consisting of the radiation oncologist, medical physicist, and radiation therapy technologist meet for an early morning conference to evaluate each patient's plan including a review of all diagnostic images that have

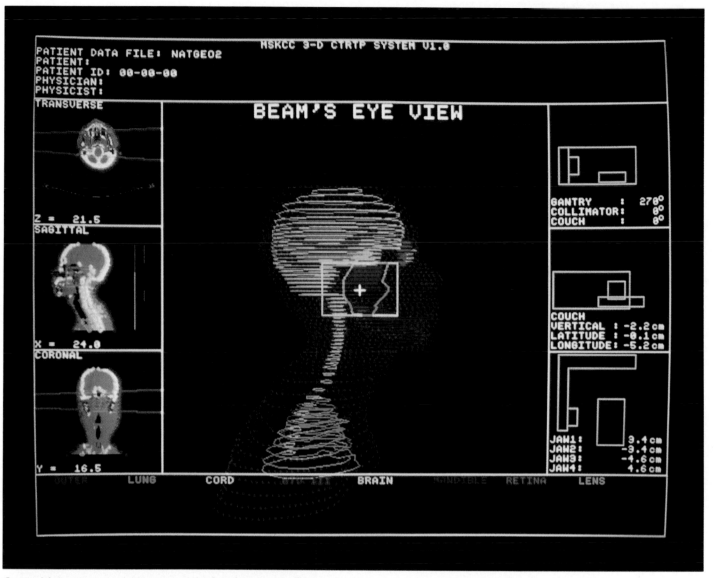

Created from dozens of CT scans of the head and neck, the exact location of a tumor is indicated by a cross mark inside the yellow box (above). This information helps to aim the radiation beams during treatment. Three views at left show different angles from which to target the tumor, while diagrams at right depict the configuration of the radiation machine as seen from the front, side and above. As the machine settings are adjusted, the diagrams change automatically. Organs sensitive to radiation such as the lungs, spinal cord, and eyes, are color-coded to help avoid unnecessary exposure.

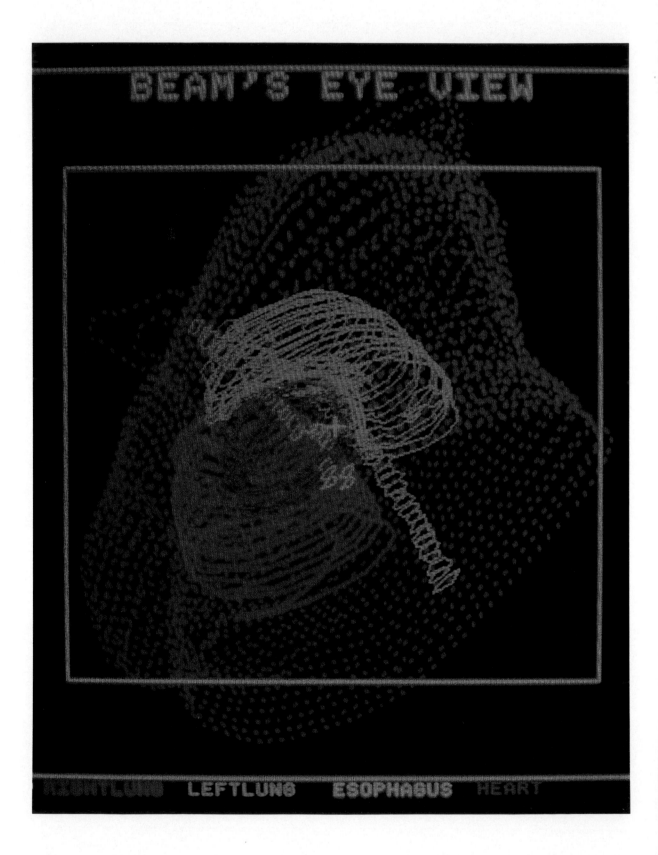

been obtained (CT, MR, US or nuclear scan), and the simulation film that duplicates the radiation beam. The patient's medical file also contains a chart that depicts the amount of radiation to be delivered and the "fallout" to organs in close proximity to the tumor.

Because 30% of cancer patients who are cured are cured by surgery, the reader may wonder why this is not the treatment of choice, but there are at least three factors that must be considered: 1), surgery is not an acceptable option in some cases. There are critical organs in the body that cannot be disabled or removed. The radiation oncologist attempts to treat the cancer with radiation while preserving the function of the organ; 2), surgery entails medical risk and is a traumatic experience, often involving extreme pain and requiring a long immobilization or recovery time. Radiation is not as traumatic and is handled on an outpatient basis; and 3), surgery sometimes results in a fallout—so called "cell showers"—that sends cancer to other parts of the body.

Finally, on many occasions radiation therapy is a valuable adjunct to surgery, and is used to shrink a tumor so that it can be surgically removed. And in most cases surgical removal of malignancies is followed by a period of radiation therapy to ensure that there is no remnant of active cancer cells that could later grow and spread.

I recalled that many of the patients previously written about—Ashleigh Slaughter, Nathan Tower, and Joe Silvers—had all been given radiation therapy as a follow-up to surgery.

Another leader in the field of radiation therapy is Dr. Robert Parker, Professor and Chairman, Department of Radiation Oncology at UCLA Medical School in Los Angeles. "I have several messages," he told me.

"At least 50% of cancer patients receive radiation therapy. The objective is cure in one half of these and we reach this objective in 40% of the cases treated for cure overall. In some cases like limited Hodgkin's disease, stage I cancer of the cervix, and skin cancer, the cure rate is 90%. In the patients we cannot cure, nearly all are helped through pain relief,

In this view of a diseased lung, it is as if the observer's eye is at the source of the radiation. What the radiation beam "sees" is illustrated by this color-coded display made at Memorial Sloan-Kettering Cancer Center in New York. Generated from many CT scans, it aids the radiation oncologist in formulating the treatment plan for cancer found in the lungs of this patient.

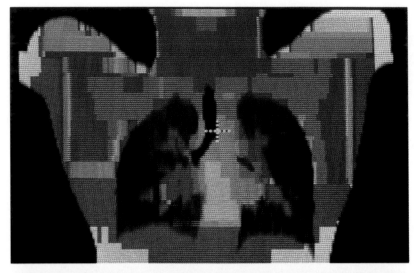

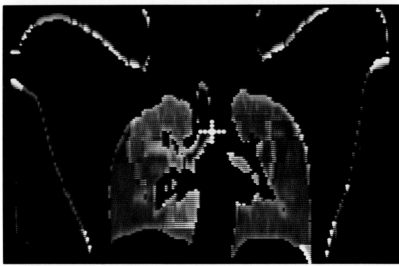

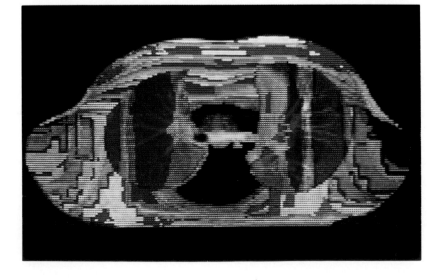

healing of open lesions, avoidance of fractures, and relief of obstructions in blood vessels or the esophagus. We can preserve the body part and function as in the eye, prostate, tongue, nose, ear, brain, spinal cord and skeleton. Radiation can be delivered with great accuracy. With the aid of CT and MR, we can achieve precise treatment."

With funds from the National Cancer Institute, Dr. Parker has set up a multi-million dollar facility close to the UCLA campus where he and his colleagues are doing pioneering work in neutron therapy. The neutron is used to bombard the cancer; its energy is different from that of the electron, photon, or proton.

Since September of 1986, up to ten patients a day receive neutron treatment which is being carefully evaluated. So far, fast neutron therapy has proved very effective with cancers of the salivary and prostate glands. It has been very effective with fast-growing and extremely slow-growing cancers, and can focus its beam to a very small volume of tissue.

With higher energy sources, the radiation oncologist hopes to use beams that are more penetrating with less damage to normal tissue.

Another expert in the use of the linear accelerator is Dr. Jay Cooper at NYU Medical Center in New York. His department treats over 100 patients daily on three machines (one cobalt and two linear accelerators). Each machine weighs as much as six tons and costs $1.5 million plus the cost of constructing a radiation-shielded room.

The expertise of the radiation oncologist lies in his knowledge of the best method of treatment for a specific tumor in a specific location. Among many other things, he must decide on total dose, time of delivery, amount and kind of radiation (electron, photon, neutron or proton), possible harm to surrounding tissue areas, and expected tumor response. "We must tailor our treatment to each patient: each is different." Dr. Cooper's average treatment plan runs from four to six weeks with a 10- to 15-minute treatment given five days a week.

Future work in improving radiation therapy, according to Dr. Cooper, lies in the continued development of chemicals that both sensitize tumors

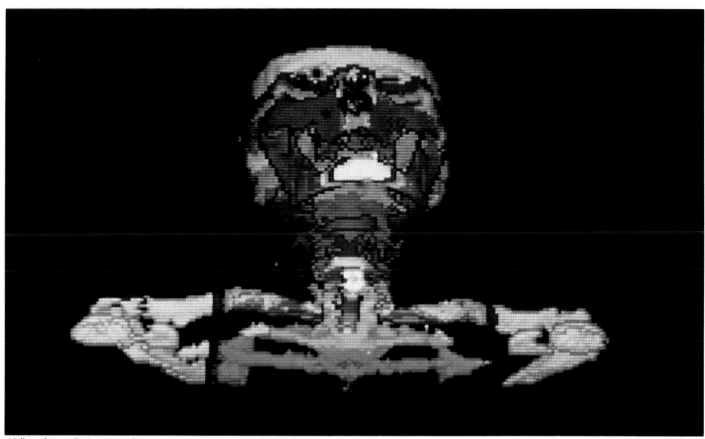

Aiding the radiation oncologist to assess the special anatomy of
each cancer patient, the distribution of radiation dose and the
exact placement of the radiation beam, more than 60 CT scans
were assembled in the case above. Cancer was in the thorax.
Fifty percent of patients with cancer receive radiation therapy.
Cure rates vary with the type and location of cancer and the
time of its detection.

Computer generated images of the lungs which
can be easily damaged by excess radiation are
used to plan treatment. Three detailed views
indicate the location of a malignancy.
Color code gives location of tumor and varying
amounts of radiation to surrounding tissues.
Computer processing of CT images subtracts
unwanted information, emphasizing details of
the tumor.

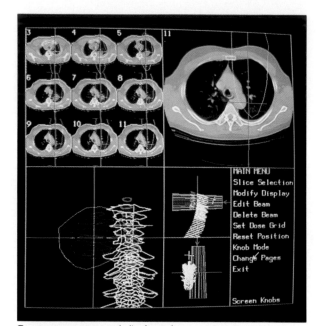

MAIN MENU
Slice Selection
Modify Display
Edit Beam
Delete Beam
Set Dose Grid
Reset Position
Knob Mode
Change Pages
Exit

Screen Knobs

Computer processed display of a tumor adjacent to the spine is viewed on a monitor. Nine axial CT sections in top left quadrant of photograph show the full dimension of the tumor from top to bottom. Top right quadrant is an enlarged view of a selected frame; lower left quadrant is a side view of the tumor in red adjacent to the spine (right); fourth quadrant indicates beam angles that can be used in treatment.

and desensitize normal tissue. Some drugs administered to cancers make them react more quickly to radiation therapy; other drugs absorbed by surrounding tissues make this healthy tissue less vulnerable to radiation.

Another area of activity is in hyperthermia where the temperature of the tumor is raised to about 42° or 43° C (about 100° F) using ultrasound, microwaves, or conduction heating. Hyperthermia has been very effective in certain types of superficial tumors and in combination with brachytherapy.

Radiation therapy equipment is also being used during surgery where larger doses can be quickly given after internal structures have been exposed by the surgeon's knife.

As in the case of MR, the medical physicist is a vital member of the radiation team. He or she offers technical support and is responsible for the precise functioning of the equipment which is frequently and carefully checked and recalibrated.

Before undergoing radiation therapy, it is important to verify the credentials of the team conducting the therapy. An MD radiation oncologist, a certified medical physicist, and an adequate number of registered therapy technologists, dosimetrists and nurses should staff any facility doing radiation therapy.

Eager to talk with a patient who had been helped by radiation therapy, I sought out a patient who had undergone treatment. Beverly Dubin is an attractive woman of 50 who looks much younger. She is married, has two children, lives in Manhattan Beach, California, and is a nurse who works with a plastic surgeon. Fully aware of the trauma and sadness in the patients she sees daily—mainly women who had radical mastectomies (breast removal)—she was emotionally devastated when, after a routine mammogram, she was told that there was a possible problem. Small calcifications in the upper and outer quadrant of a breast had been revealed by the mammogram.

A believer in early detection and earliest possible treatment, she had a biopsy performed on each breast. A 1 ½″ incision was made and samples of the tissue were removed. Several days later she received the results, ``intraductal invasive malignancy''—breast cancer in one breast.

``The surgeon recommended a radical mastectomy,'' she explained to me. ``I tried to push it out of my mind. It was mutilation of my body. I saw three other surgeons; all recommended radical mastectomy.

``I was in shock. I turned to my daughter for support, searched for an alternative, and finally talked to an oncologist at UCLA Medical Center. He told me there *was* an alternative. It was radiation therapy.''

But before proceeding, he wanted to be sure the cancer had not spread. An axillary node resection and microscopic examination indicated the cancer had not spread. ``Five days a week, for eight weeks, promptly at 4:30 PM, I went for a cobalt treatment. I didn't lose a day's work,'' Beverly told me.

Now, three years later, she has suffered no recurrence of cancer, feels good, and looks good. I asked if she had any side effects from the radiation, either during the treatment or later. She told me that there was a little soreness, a redness of the skin, and that her treated breast got a little larger temporarily (other patients told me of shrinkage).

Beverly has become an outspoken advocate of treatment of breast cancer by radiation. Certainly it is not called for in all cases, but in many cases it is an option to be considered by the patient, and her message is that surgery is not the *only* option.

``I talk to women every day who come for reconstruction after a mastectomy. Many of them could have taken the option I took and avoided the removal of their breasts.''

One of the most difficult and life-threatening procedures for a patient is cancer which lies at the base of the brain adjacent to the spinal cord. In 1983, Carol Padilla, a middle-aged mother of four children, was diagnosed as having cervical spine cancer after an MR scan. It was her second MR scan that year; the first had not defined the tumor.

Carol's health was deteriorating rapidly. She lost feeling in her left arm and leg. Surgery was recommended, and in February of 1983 a malignant

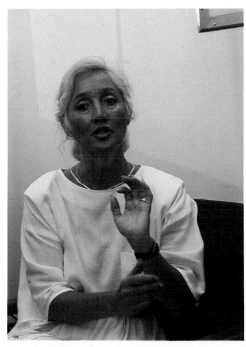

Beverly Dubin whose breast cancer was cured by radiation therapy.

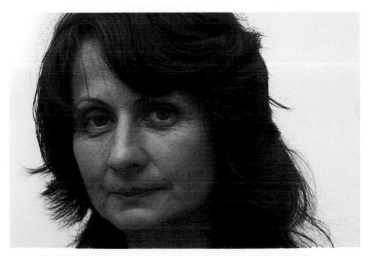

Carol Padilla whose spinal cancer was cured by radiation therapy.

tumor was partially removed from her spine in the neck at the base of the brain. Because of the danger to her spine, only 95% of the tumor was removed; even so, after surgery she couldn't walk or turn her head.

Dr. Robert Parker, who consulted on this case, knew of the new proton procedures being used experimentally at Massachusetts General Hospital in Boston. The advantage of proton therapy is the delivery of high doses to very small areas with minimum damage to surrounding tissues. Carol's problem was an exact fit for this therapy.

Carol flew to Boston with her mother where she underwent radiation therapy two days a week and later four days a week for two and a half months. The treatment did produce some side effects: she lost weight, lost her sense of taste, had a burning sensation in her throat and had difficulty swallowing food or water.

But now, four years later, she is feeling fine and is back to work as a teaching assistant in third grade classes. "I experienced a miraculous change," she assured me. She undergoes a yearly MR scan to evaluate the former tumor site.

Robert Halff is a happy bachelor approaching 80. He has led an exciting life as a newspaper editor in the Philippines, an advertising man for a New York ad agency, and a screen writer in Hollywood for Laurel and Hardy films.

In 1983 he underwent surgery for hemorrhoids. His proctologist performed a biopsy and found cancer of the skin near the anus. Brachytherapy, previously described in this chapter, was advised. He went to the UCLA Medical Center in Westwood, California.

The therapy was conducted during a one-week hospital stay. Eight needles, each filled with radioactive iridium, were inserted in the tumor near the anus. Bob was given this limited, high-dose treatment for 54 hours, and the cancer was cured. "I strongly recommend radiation treatment; it saved my life and preserved normal bowel functions," Bob said.

Another advocate of radiation treatment is Byron "Pete" Leonard, a Ph.D. in nuclear physics with a distinguished career in space science at the

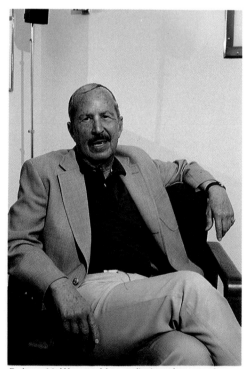

Robert Halff cured by radiation therapy for colon cancer.

Aerospace Corporation. Now 63 and semi-retired, he runs his own consulting firm.

In May of 1985 during a routine physical, his physician noted an unusual firmness in one side of the prostate gland. Cancer was later diagnosed but no symptoms were present. Pete stressed to me the enormous subtlety of the prostate cancer problem. "When you get real symptoms it's usually too late," he claimed.

With removal of the prostate you usually remove all sexual functions; so Pete, newly married to a woman eight years his junior, was worried.

A scientist with great respect for new technologies, Pete started a search for the latest information on treatment of prostate cancer. He wanted an alternative to surgery and, in all, called six doctors around the world for treatment information.

"If the average person does not avail himself of someone who understands all the subtleties in dealing with prostate cancer and does not inform himself properly, then he cannot get proper treatment. *You* must know where to go. The average doctor may not do this research. You must do it."

To make matters worse, Leonard was at a critical point in the formation of his new consulting business. "With surgery I would have been hospitalized and out of business for three weeks." He felt his business would be ruined during that time.

Armed with information gained with worldwide calls, he settled for treatment by Dr. Robert Parker at UCLA.

Radiation treatment using the linear accelerator cleared the prostate cancer. The only side effect was a temporary and slight amount of rectal bleeding. Sexual functions were preserved, and regular checkups (every three months) have disclosed no recurrence of the cancer.

Dr. Parker left another indelible thought with me about radiation therapy. "You often hear physicians and others express concern that 'radiation may cause a cancer.' In a study of 1,800 patients with head and neck cancers and another 1,200 with breast cancers, we found that the risk of cancer from radiation was no greater than the frequency of secondary cancers following surgery. We treat 1,000 patients a year

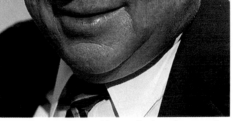

Byron Leonard cured by radiation therapy for prostate cancer.

with radiation. The risk of second cancers in adults caused by radiation should not be a factor in deciding on treatment."

"As a young medical student, I was diagnosed as having Hodgkin's disease. The cure of Hodgkin's by radiation treatment propelled me into specializing in radiation therapy."

Dr. Russel Hafer, quoted above, is a radiation oncologist at Hoag Memorial Hospital in Newport Beach, California. In 1979 while in medical school at UCLA, he noted a small mass, round and firm, beneath the skin on the right side of his neck. It was over 1" in diameter. He did little about it until he found a second mass developing in his chest. A biopsy revealed Hodgkin's disease.

Dr. Hafer knew that radiation therapy had a 90% cure rate for his stage of disease and he opted

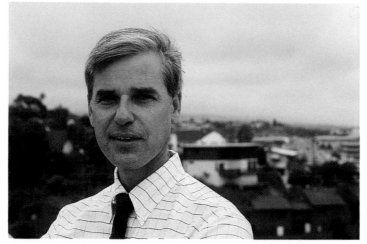

Russel Hafer, M.D., cured by radiation therapy for chest cancer.

for this therapy. For five weeks, he underwent five treatments a week at UCLA. He has had no recurrence and is happily married with two children.

Catherine L. St. Clair is an articulate, 24-year-old librarian in Corona Del Mar, California. In 1980, at age 16, she started to have memory lapses: she would lose her car in a parking lot, and couldn't remember her homework assignments. She slept a lot, suffered from extreme fatigue, and finally dropped out of school.

In December 1980, a CT scan revealed a walnut-sized cyst in the brain just above the pituitary gland. Surgery was performed and 90% of the cyst was removed. Postsurgical infection resulted—both meningitis and osteomyelitis—and part of the cranial bone became infected in the area of the original surgery. A second operation was performed in February of 1981 to remove the infected bone.

In July of 1982, a CT scan revealed that the tumor had reappeared. A third operation, a craniotomy, was performed in August of 1982, but the tumor couldn't be reached transnasally. In a fourth operation in January 1983, a catheter was inserted into the brain in an attempt to remove the cyst, but the gelatinous tissue of which it was formed was too thick and could not be withdrawn.

After three unsuccessful operations, Catherine turned to radiation therapy. Treatment began in the spring of 1983. Five days a week for five weeks she went to UCLA Medical Center for radiation therapy, each treatment lasting just one minute.

Since completion of her radiation treatment in April 1983, she has had no recurrence of the cyst; this is confirmed by yearly CT scans.

Catherine faults herself for not having started with radiation therapy, but says that the whole experience has been very valuable. "Our family has drawn more closely together. I know the value of life and am not going to waste mine. I have sorted things out and now know what I really want, what is really important."

Ken Heitz, now 40, a successful lawyer with a wife and two children, was a star on the UCLA Varsity Basketball Team and played in three national championships.

In October 1985, he was at Harvard University recruiting young lawyers for his firm. During an early morning jog, he accidently discovered a small lump just above his left knee. He was very busy interviewing for the firm, traveled constantly, and neglected the growing lump.

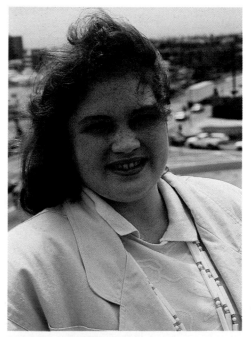

Catherine L. St. Clair cured by radiation therapy for a brain tumor.

Four months later, while playing tennis, the lump became painful and the leg started throbbing. Ken was frightened and went to see his old friend and athletic trainer at UCLA, "Ducky Drake." Drake pushed and probed the lump, became concerned, and sent him to the UCLA team physician, Dr. Todd Grant. Within two hours he underwent CT scanning at nearby St. John's Hospital. CT showed a lime-sized cyst and a biopsy confirmed a liposarcoma—an active, malignant tumor.

In the recent past, Ken Heitz' leg would have been amputated. Instead he chose a treatment called the UCLA Limb Salvage. In the first phase of this three-part procedure, the tumor is precisely located, a catheter is inserted and drips a toxic drug (usually adriamycin) into the tumor, and a bolus of contrast material is sent through the catheter revealing the dispersal of the drug at the tumor site. For 72 hours, Ken watched the adriamycin drip into the tumor. Immediately after the catheter was removed, he underwent five days of radiation therapy (the second phase).

In the third phase of the protocol, surgery was performed to remove the tumor. Since treatment, Ken has had checkups to see if the tumor metastasized (spread); it has not.

"My great fortune was in having the UCLA connection," Ken felt. "It was a real miracle. I still jog, ski, play tennis and basketball. Six months after the treatment, I shot a basket."

Here again, radiation therapy used with limited surgery had proved to be a highly successful alternative to amputation.

The previous seven case studies are examples of what the best of modern radiation therapy can accomplish. In the United States, many patients are cured of cancer by radiation therapy every year, but the technique does involve risks. Many patients suffer such temporary side effects as nausea, diarrhea, burning sensations, and hair loss.

But the risk/reward ratio is so high and the negatives are so few that each year more and more patients are turning to radiation therapy as an alternative to extensive surgery.

Dr. Eli Glatstein, a self-described curmudgeon and skeptic, heads the Radiation Oncology Branch at

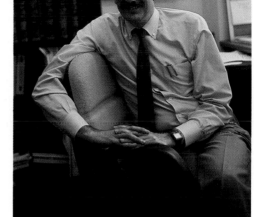

Ken Heitz cured by radiation therapy for a tumor in his leg.

the National Cancer Institute in Bethesda, Maryland. He is a world-renowned expert on radiation therapy, and I asked about new areas of research in the field.

He told me about studies of different types of energy: helium ions, pions, neutrons, and protons. Each is being evaluated to determine what part they can play in the destruction of cancer cells.

He told me, too, about radiation sensitizers (IUDR and BUDR) that make cancer cells more receptive to treatment, and radiation protectors (WR 2721) that "shield" healthy cells during radiation treatment.

In another research activity (photodynamic therapy), light generated by gold vapor or argon lasers is absorbed by the hematoporphyrin in the cancer cell, and in the process of absorption the cell is killed. Normal cells do not contain hematoporphyrin and are spared.

To the layman, radiation therapy has been a mysterious and little understood component in the battle against cancer. Today, however, it plays an important role in treatment and cure, and has great potential for more successful applications in the future.

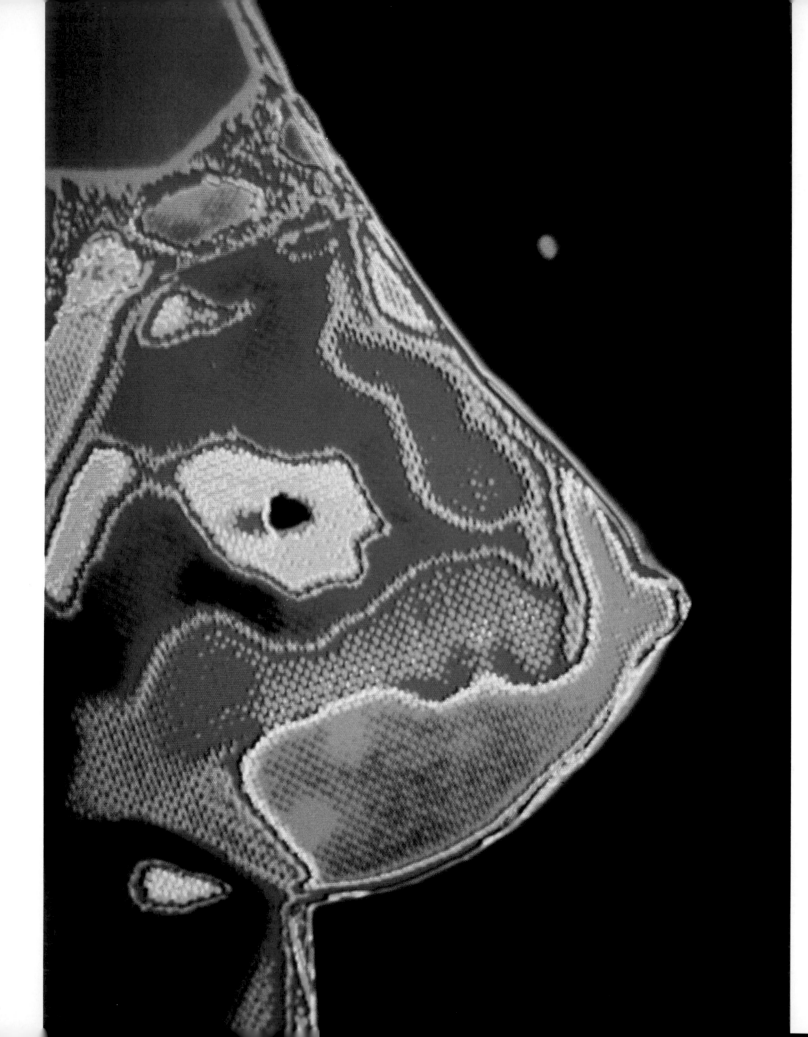

VII. MAMMOGRAPHY

"Please, please go and have a yearly mammogram" —NANCY REAGAN

Breast cancer will develop in one out of ten women in their lifetime. Six million new cases will be diagnosed, and over 42,000 women will die this year making breast cancer a leading cancer killer of women today. Statistics show that with early detection by mammography, almost one-third of these fatalities could have been prevented. Yet, in spite of this, fewer than 20% of women over age 50 (when frequency of breast cancer is the highest) have an annual breast exam.

When asked why they don't have a regular mammogram, most women will blame their fear of radiation or simply say, "my doctor didn't suggest it." With greater education about the negligible radiation exposure and growing physician awareness, more women each year undergo mammography screening and practice self-examination. Recently, when the President's wife Nancy Reagan was diagnosed as having breast cancer after a routine mammogram, one breast imaging clinic reported a 50% increase in patients requesting the screening.

Breast cancer is any malignant growth in the tissue of the breast; its cause is unknown. Without warning, cells begin to grow abnormally and often spread to other areas of the body. There are many types of breast cancer, and tumors in one part of the breast are different from tumors in another. Some grow fast, others take years to develop; some are

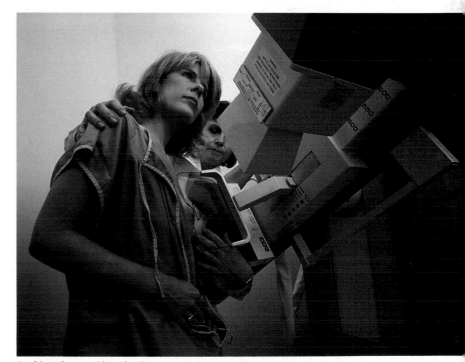

Lurking deep within the lobes and ducts of the breast, abnormal cells are detected by mammographic screening. In the color enhanced image to the left (side view of a breast) the small black dot surrounded by a contour of colors indicates a malignancy. Above, a technologist positions a patient for a screening exam. No abnormality was found. Breast cancer is best treated when detected early.

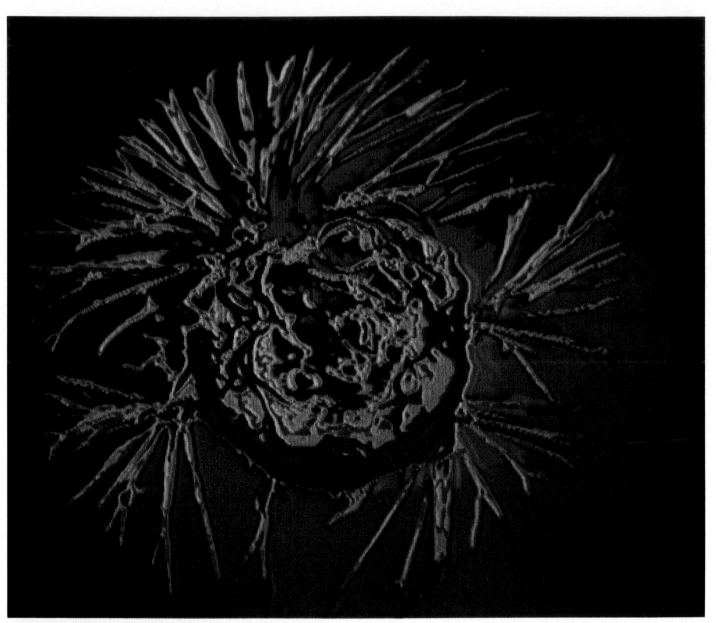

A remarkable electron microscope view of a single cancer cell removed from the breast of a patient at the National Institutes of Health in Bethesda, Maryland shows ``tentacles'' reaching out from the cell's central core. The word cancer is derived from the Greek word for crab. These cells make up what is called a stellate lesion found in the breasts of women who are usually over 50 years old.

microscopic and may never pose a threat while others can be large and quickly become life-threatening.

Eighty-five percent of breast cancers found by mammography can be treated either surgically, by radiation therapy, with chemotherapy, or any combination of the three. Unfortunately, about half of the women with breast cancer find out too late that it has spread to other areas of the body.

After it has become wide spread, control may be achieved with chemotherapy, but cure is unlikely. Early detection and treatment are the keys to curing breast cancer.

The breast is a glandular organ. It has 15 to 20 tree-like lobes. Each lobe has 100 or so tiny bulbs or acini where milk is produced. During lactation, milk flows from the acini into the lobes, then through ducts to the surface of the breast at the nipple. The lobes, ducts, and acini are surrounded by fat which comprises most of the breast. The entire gland is enclosed in a membrane called the fascia.

The lymphatic system is the route by which breast cancer spreads. The lymph nodes are part of the body's immune system and contain a high concentration of white blood cells. Lymph fluid bathes the body cells and fights off disease. Breast tissue is drained by lymphatic vessels that lie in the spaces between and around the milk-producing lobes. These vessels lead to clusters of lymph nodes in the armpits and along the breastbone.

Cancer cells from the breast often spread to the lymph nodes. When this happens, the lymph nodes become large and hard. The breast cancer diagnostic procedure often includes biopsy of the lymph nodes to determine if cancer cells are present.

Mammography, as performed by radiologists in facilities with specially trained technologists and state-of-the-art x-ray equipment, is the most reliable method of detecting breast cancer even before it can be felt by self-examination or by a doctor's palpation.

The equipment used in mammography is specially designed to image breast tissues which are soft and of uniform density. Very subtle changes must be identified in very fine detail including extremely small areas of calcification. The radiation

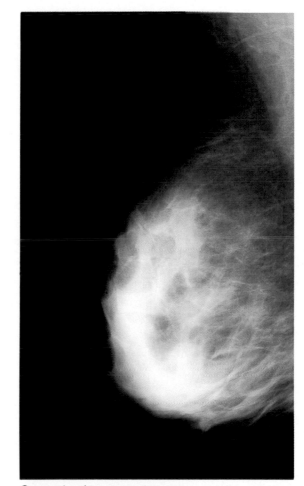

Conventional x-ray can detect an abnormal mass. Nearly 20 million mammograms are done annually in the U.S., but 80% of the female population ignores the test that could be life-saving.

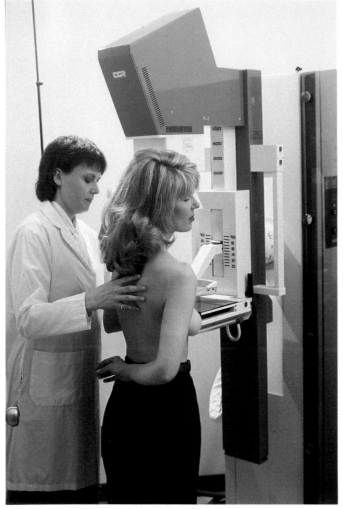

In a standard exam, a plastic plate compresses or flattens the breast to obtain better detail of its entire area. The procedure is fast, painless, and requires a minimal amount of radiation.

dose must, of course, be kept to a minimum.

The most up-to-date mammographic equipment consists of a large control box (2′ × 3′ × 5′), voltage generators (20 to 50 kilovolts) and an adjustable x-ray unit that can be raised, lowered, and rotated to conform to the height and physical characteristics of the patient.

The patient undresses from the waist up and slips on a gown. The test is quick and painless. Each breast is x-rayed in two or three views. The patient usually stands next to the machine and—with the assistance of a technologist—places a single breast on a film plate beneath the x-ray tube. A padded compression plate is lowered from above and gently squeezes the breast to facilitate better imaging of the entire breast. The patient is told to hold her breath as views are taken of each breast.

The film is processed immediately while the patient waits in the mammography area or anteroom. If the technologist is pleased with the film exposure, sharpness of the image, and area coverage, the patient is sent home to await the radiologist's report. The radiation dose is extremely low.

Besides the film approach described above, a second type of imaging technique is used. This procedure produces an electrostatic image on paper and is called xeroradiography or xeromammography. Both techniques produce comparable results in terms of diagnostic accuracy. The choice of one over the other depends on the radiologist's preference.

The key player in any story about mammography is the radiologist and his or her function is the interpretation of the films. One radiologist described reading mammograms as ''dancing on the head of a needle many times a day.''

Breast cancer can be treated by surgery, radiation therapy, or a combination of both. This view of a radiation therapist's screen serves as a treatment guide for radiation therapy.
At the left of the screen are various anatomical views. The center screen is a view as seen from the source of radiation. The right three views indicate equipment positioning.
Many women opt for radiation therapy since it preserves the size and shape of the breast and does not require hospitalization. With early detection approx. 75% of all breast cancer patients can be saved.

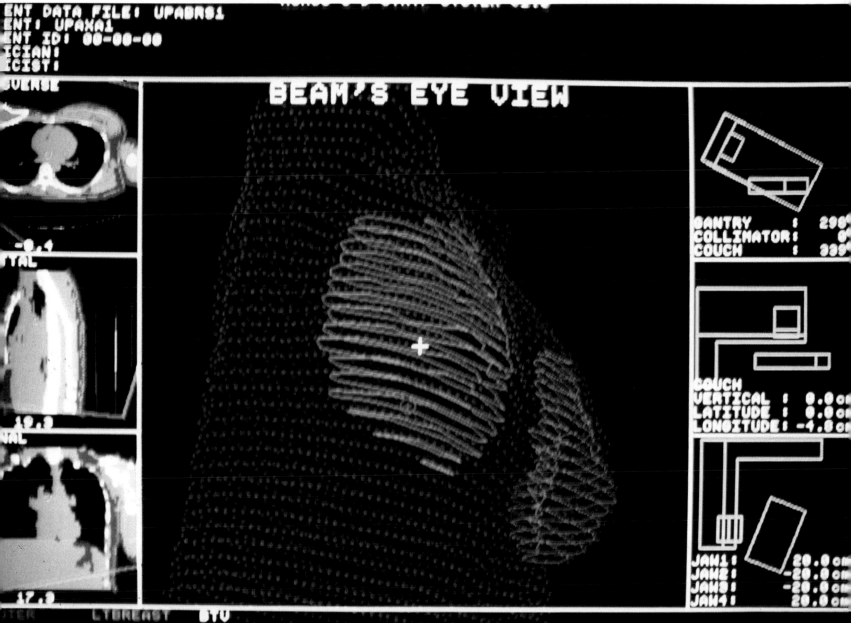

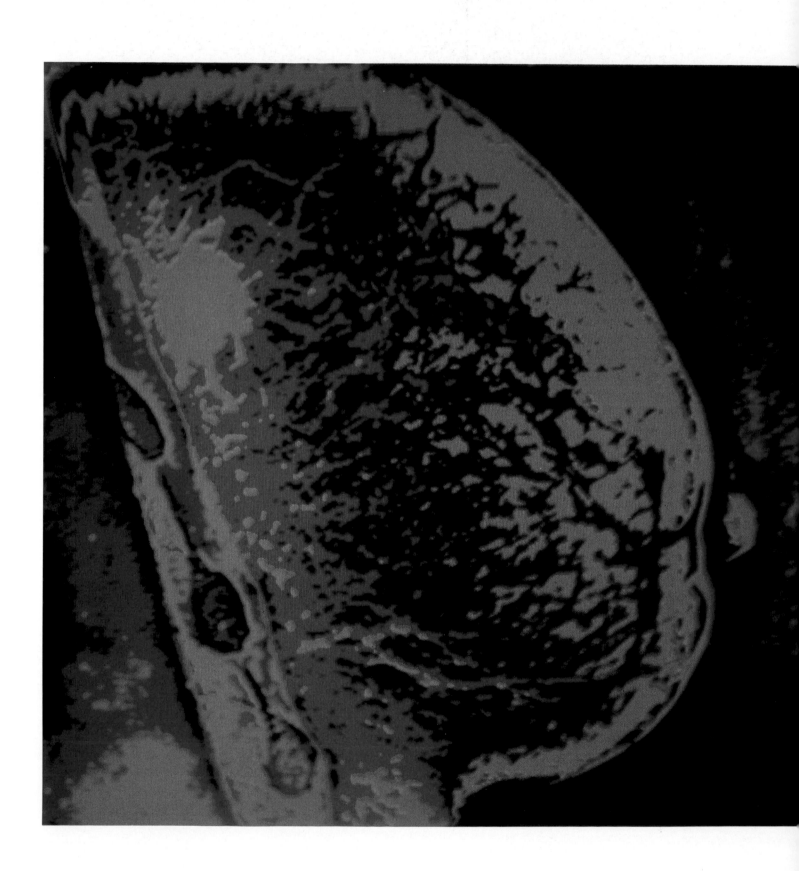

To get a first hand idea of just how difficult (but very rewarding) the film interpretation process can be, I traveled to Rochester, New York to spend a day with Dr. Wende W. Logan, one of the busiest mammographers in the country. Her patients call her "Eagle Eye" for her ability to see things that others cannot. In a maze of tiny rooms in a long central corridor, Dr. Logan and her staff of 35 highly-trained technologists perform breast examinations on 100 to 150 patients daily. Each of seven x-ray units, meticulously maintained and checked for radiation levels, are used to screen about 15 patients an hour. Dr. Logan personally evaluates every x-ray film.

In 1986, the last year for which she has comprehensive data, 20,000 patients were imaged; of these, 292 had positive cancers. Yet as expert as she is, Dr. Logan admits that she missed or did not find the cancer in 4% of her patients. In 1988 she will see over 30,000 patients and it is probable that about 400 will have malignancies, 320 of these will be saved by surgery and/or radiation therapy, and about 80 cases will be fatal.

There are many kinds of breast cancers, Dr. Logan told me. Some are as small as fine grains of sand that "pepper" an area in the breast. Others are huge, calcified tumors over 1" in diameter. Between these extremes are lesions of many kinds, tumors both hard and soft, and cysts that are sacs or pouches containing fluid-like matter. Mammographers further categorize lesions into circumscribed (blob-like and multishaped) and stellate (shaped like a star). The latter have a "sunburst" appearance with uneven, tentacle-like arms radiating from a central mass.

Dr. Logan is expert in a technique called "needle aspiration." Her first patient of the day needed such a procedure. Referred to Dr. Logan by her family doctor, the patient had a large cyst in her left breast. The referring physician had recommended surgery, but the patient wanted a

The pink area in this breast near the chest wall is malignant. A mastectomy was performed on this patient after detection. She is still alive ten years after surgery; no other cancer has been detected.

second opinion from "Eagle Eye." On observing the old x-rays that the patient brought with her and new x-rays obtained that day, Dr. Logan recognized that the lump was a benign, liquid-filled sac. In a procedure that took about five minutes, Dr. Logan carefully inserted a needle into the mass, removed the fluid from the cyst, and sent it to a pathologist for study. No cancer existed, and a mastectomy was avoided.

Dr. Logan is a bundle of energy: at one moment she is examining films in her viewing room, the next she is consulting with a patient who "must personally see her." She spends time with anyone who wants to see her even if their films show no sign of disease.

Just before noon, an elderly lady with tears in her eyes slowly moved down the corridor with her cane. Dr. Logan had diagnosed breast cancer some weeks earlier and a lumpectomy was performed.

"I just wanted to personally thank you," she told Dr. Logan. "I feel great, now." Dr. Logan threw her arms around the patient and kissed her. "You look fine, kid," she said. "Come back and see me in a year."

Reading a mammogram accurately is a matter of visual perception and clinical skills, plus years of experience. Since about 10% of lesions do not show up on mammograms, physical examination by a physician is always necessary.

While looking at some films with Dr. Logan, I noticed a huge, half-moon area on one patient's film. "My lord, what's that?" I asked. "Oh, those are silicon implants," Dr. Logan told me, "breast builders. They sure make the detection of cancer more difficult."

Dr. Logan explained that silicon is radiopaque, and tissue that could be cancerous might be hidden in front of or behind the implant. In the past, it was discovered that liquid silicon injected into the breasts for cosmetic reasons could cause cancer; the new implants, however, do not of themselves produce cancer.

Dr. Logan advises that the most important thing for a woman over 50 is to get a "baseline" (first) mammogram. "Don't play ostrich with your life and your health."

Mrs. Margaret Spellman reads quietly in her home near Rochester, New York. A mammogram disclosed a lump in her right breast. She prepared for surgery but a simple procedure called ``needle aspiration,'' wherein a small hollow needle literally drains the lump, was used. ``You can't believe this,'' she told me, ``but the lump just disappeared.''

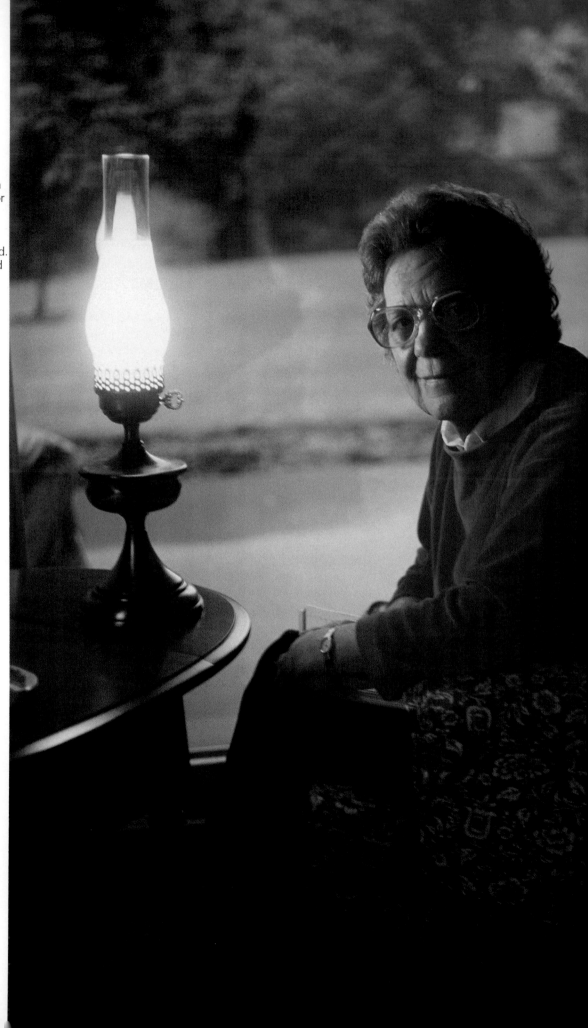

Mrs. Margaret Spellman, at 76, is a gracious woman who radiates the charm and hospitality of a bygone era. Though active and happy, she has had a series of medical problems during the past few years that required quadruple bypass surgery, skin cancer surgery, and cataract surgery on her left eye.

During a routine physical, her family doctor felt a lump in her right breast. He referred her to Dr. Logan for a mammogram.

"At first I was taken aback when I met her; pigtails, white tennis shirt, dark jeans—not like a doctor at all," Mrs. Spellman reminisced about Dr. Logan.

"But I found her to be a very casual person of great personal warmth. She called me in to show me my x-rays mounted on a light box on her wall. I could see a spot on the right breast. She did an ultrasound scan to confirm the information on the x-ray, and it also imaged a cyst in the same area."

"My mother had breast cancer and went through with a radical mastectomy. I was frightened and immediately prepared for surgery, but Dr. Logan did a second series of mammograms and decided to do a needle aspiration. During a following visit a new set of films showed that the lump had disappeared."

Five years have passed since Mrs. Spellman's first exam. She has had no complications and makes a yearly visit to Dr. Logan to verify there is no regrowth of "those nasty lumps."

Eleanor Rink is a tall, attractive, middle-aged woman of 48, who has a handsome husband and three beautiful daughters. One day her best friend and neighbor asked her to come along for moral support as she drove from her home in Hornell, New York to see Dr. Logan for a mammogram. During the hour long drive, Eleanor decided she too would have a mammogram.

After the study was completed and evaluated, Dr. Logan called her in and broke the bad news: "There is something that isn't right. I feel a thickening. Don't panic, but do something about it this week."

Mrs. Rink went to a surgeon that week and

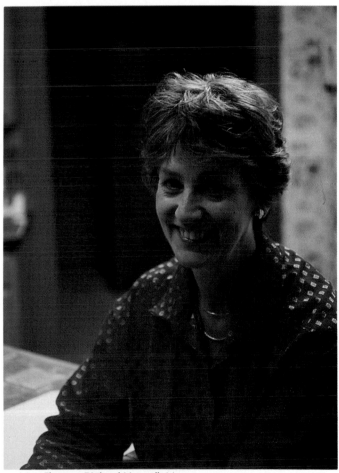

Mrs. Eleanor Rink of Hornell, New York accompanied a friend for a screening mammogram, decided to undergo one herself, and the radiologist discovered cancer. She chose a minimal surgical procedure called a lumpectomy followed by radiation therapy on her left breast. "Without a mammogram, I wouldn't be here today," she explained.

three days later a biopsy was performed. The results indicated a malignant tumor.

She consulted with many people and found she had several options: a lumpectomy to remove the tumor, a modified mastectomy to remove the tumor and surrounding tissue, or a radical mastectomy to remove the entire breast, muscle tissue, and underarm lymph glands. Radiation therapy was suggested as another alternative.

Eleanor agonized over the decision. She called Dr. Logan several times at home and always found her helpful and patient—"doing whatever she could to help me work out the problem."

Finally, with great understanding and support from her husband and daughters, Mrs. Rink opted for a lumpectomy with radiation therapy as follow-up treatment. A second biopsy of Eleanor's lymph nodes showed no spread of cancer. The tumor was removed, and for five weeks, five days a week, Eleanor reported to a Rochester hospital for radiation treatments.

Her odyssey began with mammography on June 20th, proceeded with surgery on July 15th, and—by September 20th—she was finished with radiation therapy.

Now, her left breast is just slightly smaller because of tissue removal, and she returns for follow-up mammograms every six months.

Eleanor told me her breast at first lost elasticity due to the radiation, was red and inflamed, then later turned brown. Today, however, it has completely returned to its original color and softness.

Her messages: 1), get a mammogram; 2), examine your options; 3), there is really no pain or discomfort; and 4), get an expert second opinion.

After my talk with Eleanor, I talked privately with her husband, Bob, who had been very supportive during this period.

"Eleanor is still not totally over the experience," he told me. "There is great anxiety every time she goes for an exam. She thinks, 'where is it going to be next time?' She remembers one day in Dr. Logan's office sitting next to a woman who was a survivor of Hitler's death camps. Eleanor got great consolation from her philosophy of survival: The woman told her, 'You must persist, you must prevail.' "

"Now my three girls, ages 23, 21 and 17, want to know when they should have their first mammogram. Our physician has advised that they should wait until they are at least 30."

In May of 1986, during routine self-examination, Arlene Riola discovered a lump quite close to the surface on the right side of her right breast. She was particularly concerned because five of the seven children in her mother's family had died from cancer.

Her family gynecologist examined her, thought it was a cyst, and sent her to see Dr. Logan.

Dr. Logan did a needle aspiration and sent the sample to a pathologist. The report came back positive. A second needle aspiration was done by Dr. Logan for confirmation, and it too indicated malignancy.

Arlene was faced with three choices: lumpectomy, modified mastectomy, or radical mastectomy.

After endless consultation, she opted for lumpectomy, radiation therapy, and brachytherapy.

Two weeks after the lumpectomy was done on an outpatient basis, she started radiation treatments. She had 23 two-minute treatments over a period of five weeks.

After eight days she was admitted to the hospital for implant radiation therapy. During a period of 34 hours, five needles filled with radio-isotopes were placed in contact with the exact area of the removed cyst. There was no pain involved, but some aftereffects such as initial tenderness, extreme reddening, and hardening of the breast tissue. "In my case," Arlene told me, "needle aspiration saved my life. I feel very fortunate."

Arlene was an offset press operator, a printer by profession. After 15 years, she had become a master in her trade, but her close call with breast cancer has changed that.

"I wanted to give something back," she told me. "My experience forced me to look at my values. It was interesting to see how people treat you and how they feel about you when you have cancer. Some people back off, they feel they will be affected. The people who help you through, and boy do you need them, are just wonderful. Your

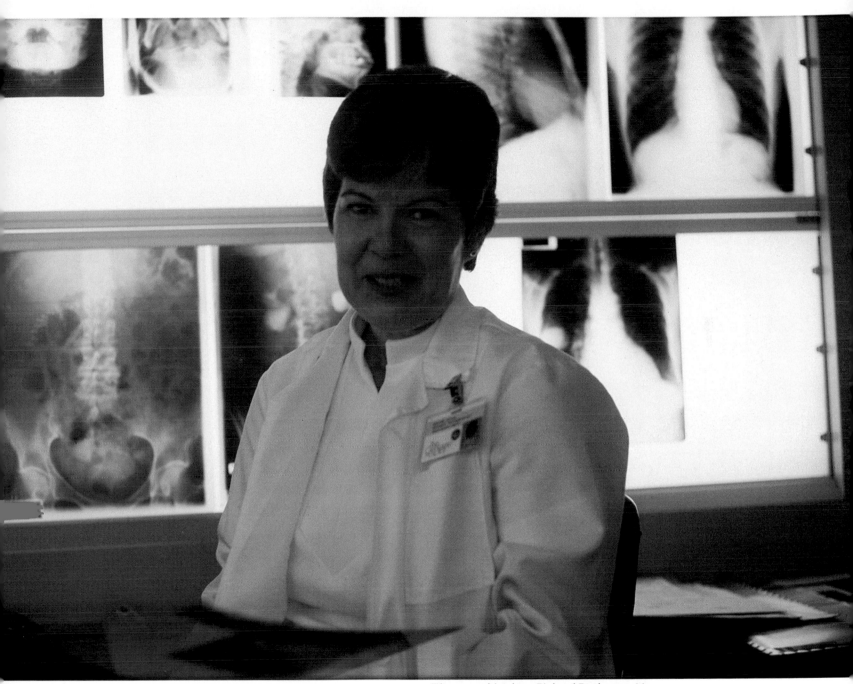

attitude toward treatment is very important. It must be positive. Don't put your head in the sand. Don't feel that this is the end of your life. What is being done today with breast cancer is phenomenal.''

Today, because Arlene Riola wanted to ''give something back,'' she has enrolled in a two-year course at Genesee Hospital to become an x-ray technologist. Her experience with breast cancer has changed her way of looking at life. It is even changing her career.

Fifty-year-old Arlene Riola of Rochester, New York was so influenced by her own experience with breast cancer that she has begun a two-year course in x-ray technology to help others who have cancer. Arlene was treated by needle aspiration, lumpectomy, and radiation therapy. Having survived, ''I would like to give something back,'' she stated.

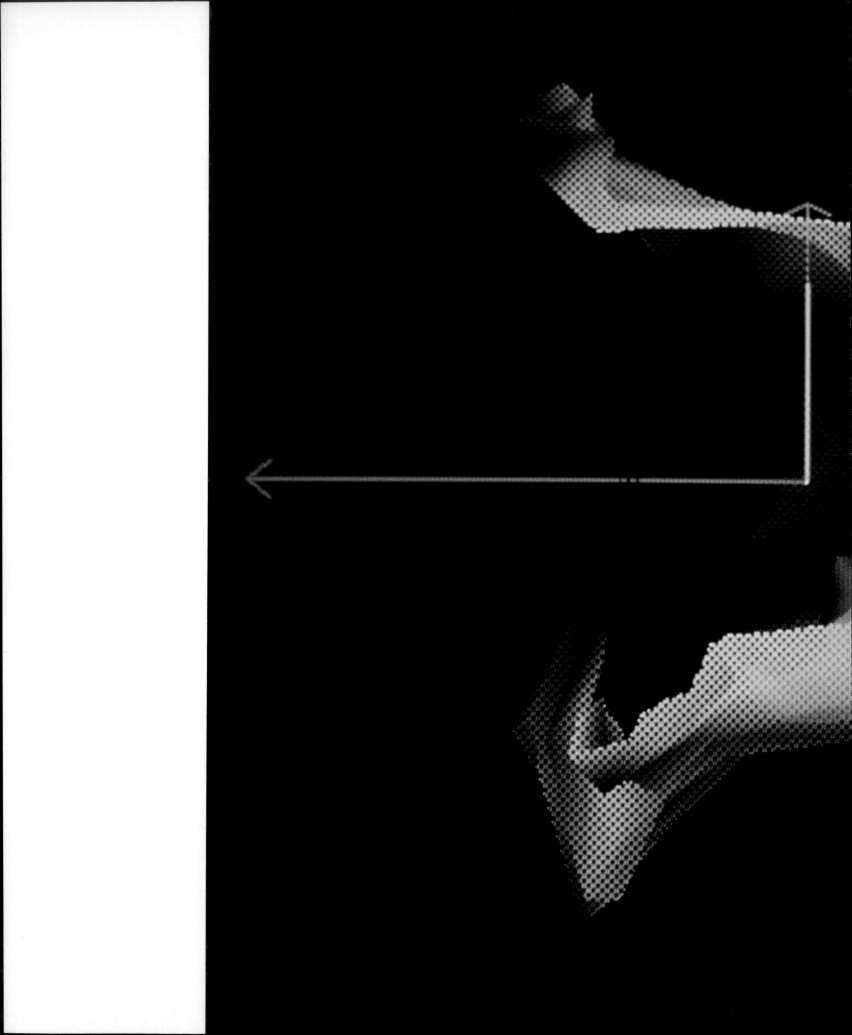

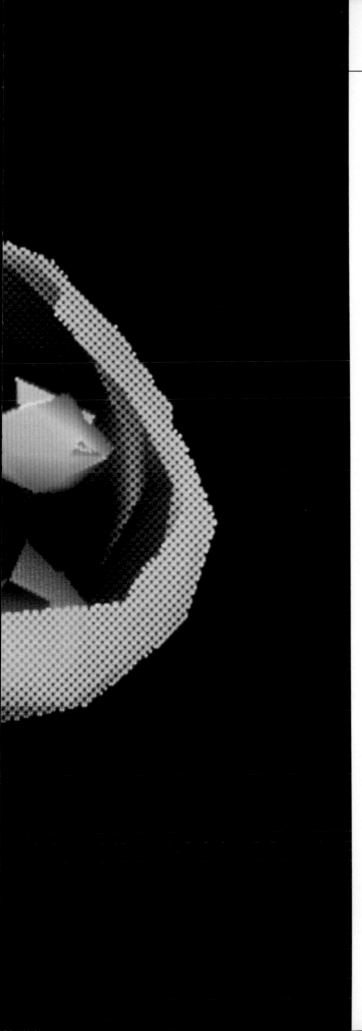

In the old days, there was an oft repeated statement by examining physicians about breast palpation: "If I can't feel it, it doesn't exist."

The work of such eminent radiologists as Jacob Gershon-Cohen at Albert Einstein Medical Center in Philadelphia did much to change that attitude. Today, we know that the primary contribution of radiology to breast cancer diagnosis and treatment is that it allows the physician to see things that *cannot* be felt.

Some common cancers take about seven years to grow to a size that can be felt. Since mammography can detect tiny cancerous growths no bigger than a grain of sand, we can now remove the malignancy and offer the patient treatment before significant health risks arise.

One of the first and still practicing mammographers in the profession is Dr. Herman C. Zuckerman. A charming, informal man pushing 75, he dresses impeccably in color-coordinated shirt and tie, and never wears the traditional white coat of his profession. A master of one-liners, he told me that "after examining 1,600,000 breasts, I'd give anything to examine just one behind!"

One evening, after he had seen the last of the 80 patients he examines daily (his appointments are backed up for two months), Dr. Zuckerman reminisced about his profession and experience.

In preparation for radiation therapy, the shape and position of a malignant tumor are accurately displayed on a monitor. Arrow depicts course of accelerator treatment beam. Lesions or tumors may be as small as a grain of sand or as massive as a large stone. After treatment the breast is often red and inflamed and the skin takes on a leathery consistency. This disappears in a few months.

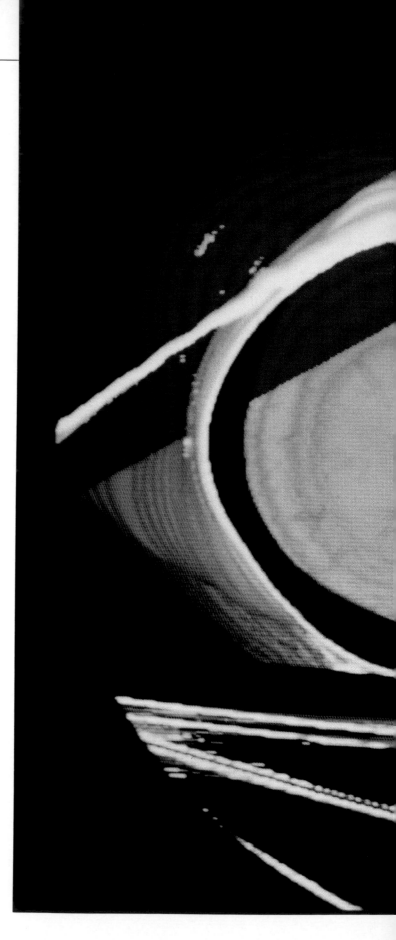

What was most interesting to me as a layman was how relatively new mammography is and how difficult it was to prove its efficacy and gain acceptance of its use.

As a young radiologist, Dr. Zuckerman attended the annual meeting of the Radiological Society of North America in Chicago in 1953. In the scientific exhibit section, he found a display of 100 foggy, cellophane-wrapped breast films that had been assembled by Dr. Jacob Gershon-Cohen.

"I couldn't make anything out of them. I examined them for six hours until the lights went out, then tipped a guard $5 to keep the lights on until 9 PM; another three hours. The next day I came back to view the films for another six hours, tipping the guard two cartons of cigarettes."

Dr. Zuckerman, whose practice was then confined to skeletal radiology, knew from viewing these early mammograms that if just one in ten women could be saved by early cancer detection, it would be far more rewarding than what he was then doing.

From 1954 to 1961, while continuing his bone work, he examined 250 women with potential breast disease who had been referred to him by surgeons. No charge was made. New x-ray machines had to be developed for this work with lower voltages and less radiation dose. He tried new industrial films, image intensifiers, film-screen systems, and experimented with development time and temperature—all the technical improvements required to get better resolution and detail.

Axial view prepared from CT scans is color-coded to indicate the amount of radiation falling on breast and lungs. In the latest technology a series of movable metal shutters are used between the energy source and patient to direct beams only to affected areas. By directing focused radiation from different angles, minimum exposure is given to healthy tissues, maximum exposure to areas of disease. Detection of cancers in patients with breast implants has proved difficult.

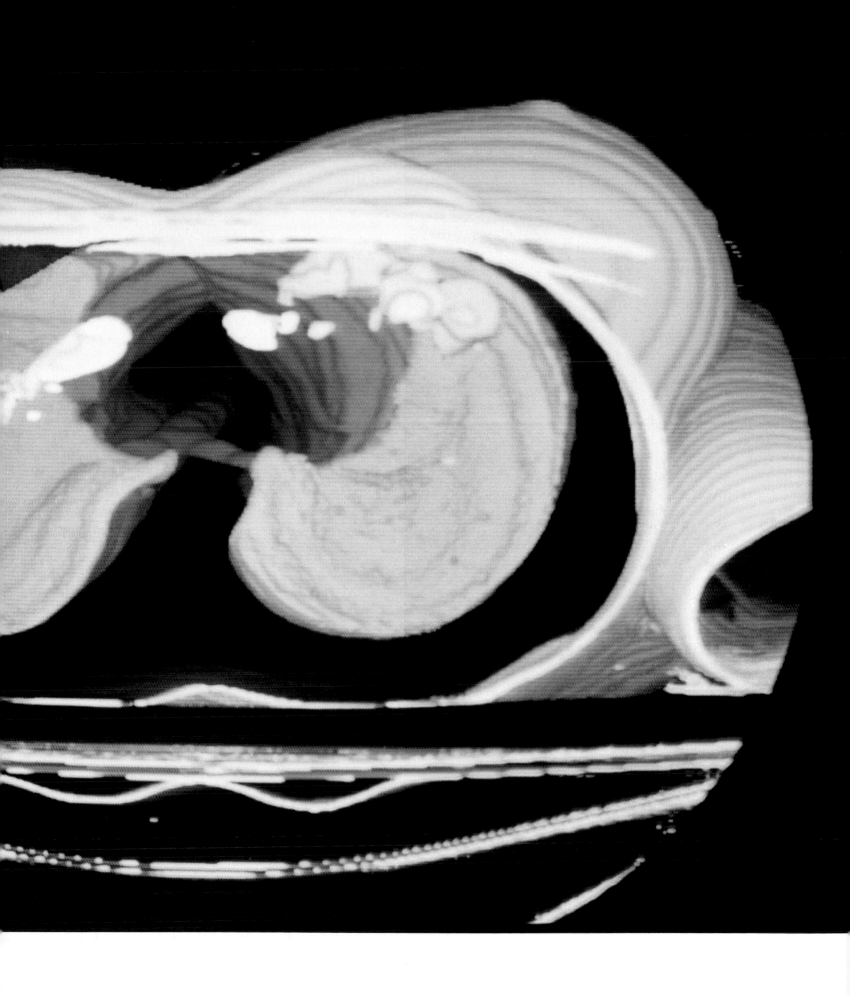

Dr. Zuckerman told me that today, "93% of breast cancer patients can be saved if you pick it up before they feel it. I started compression of the breast for mammography in 1954. Now it is routine procedure and is done for many reasons: less radiation is required; there is no overlapping of inner tissue; there is no movement of the breast during exposure; it brings the breast closer to the film; and increases the density of lesions which are not compressible."

Dr. Zuckerman reads 480 films a day (6 views, 80 patients). Until recently, he rose at 4 AM and finished dictation at 7 AM. All urgent evaluation reports are phoned to the referring physician by 9 AM on the morning following the exam. Most of the patients are alerted to a problem if it exists at the time of the exam, but it is Dr. Zuckerman's policy to have the referring physician counsel the patient about any necessary action or follow-up. Six technologists operate five x-ray machines in his busy New York office.

He continues to experiment on new and better methods of breast imaging, and has developed a 3-D system for viewing images. Much like the "stereopair" viewers of yesteryear, two images made 6° apart are exposed under the x-ray unit. They are then viewed in a special viewing box to give image dimension. This procedure is done on two or three patients daily who have specific types of breast abnormalities.

Dr. Zuckerman places great emphasis on relaxing and comforting his patients. Women coming for a breast examination are very concerned and uptight. They have been referred to Dr. Zuckerman because their physician or surgeon is checking up on a possible problem.

On one occasion, a particularly difficult patient, frustrated and concerned during the palpation asked, "Are you the doctor?"

A weary Herman Zuckerman answered: "No, I'm the electrician."

The woman stormed out to the receptionist and complained: "I've been here 2½ hours and haven't once seen the doctor." The receptionist asked if she hadn't been examined by the doctor. "No. I was examined by the electrician," she maintained.

"The more you can relax the patient the more you improve the quality of the image," Dr. Zuckerman remarked. "And remember, with breast cancer you remain a patient for the rest of your life."

As I left Dr. Zuckerman's spacious office with his newly installed viewing apparatus that holds 750 films on a rotating, motor-driven track, I spotted a beautifully engraved silver plaque on the wall. It read simply:

A message of thanks . . .
for the future you have saved for me.

Composite, computer-generated, color-coded image of mammogram and body profile delineates an area of malignancy in red. Of 400,000 detected breast cancers annually, 80% are cured and 20% prove fatal. Breast cancer accounts for 26% of all types of cancer occurring in women.

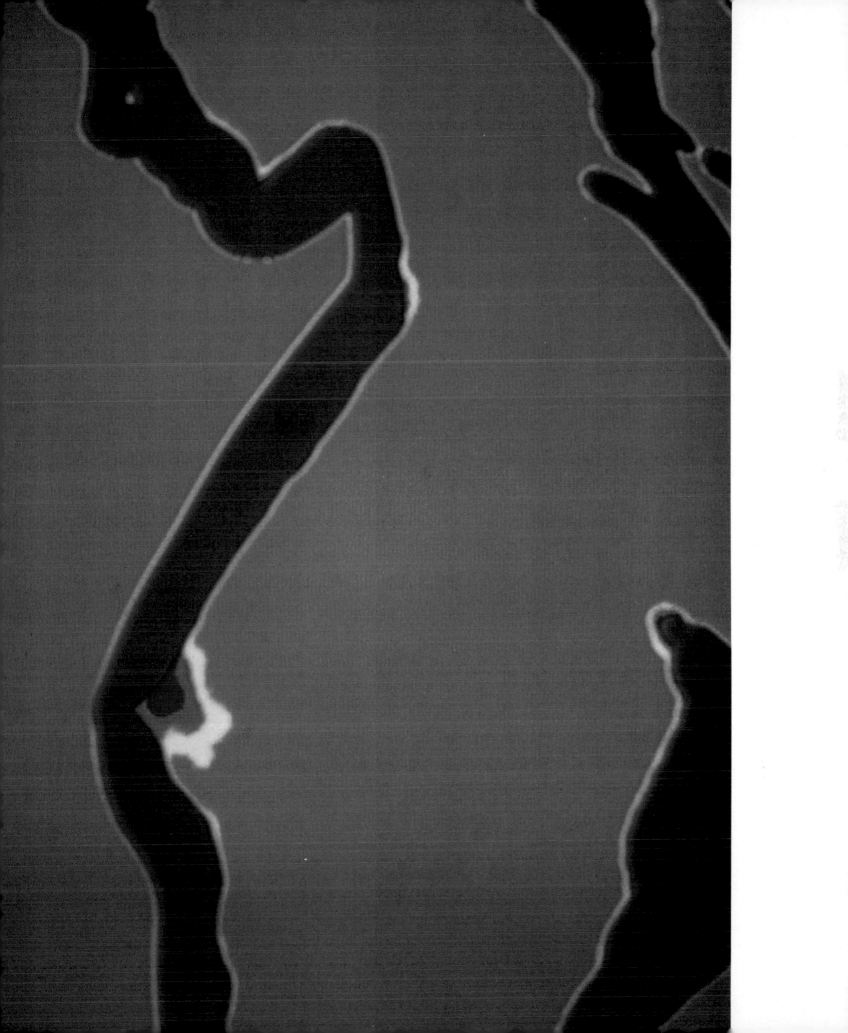

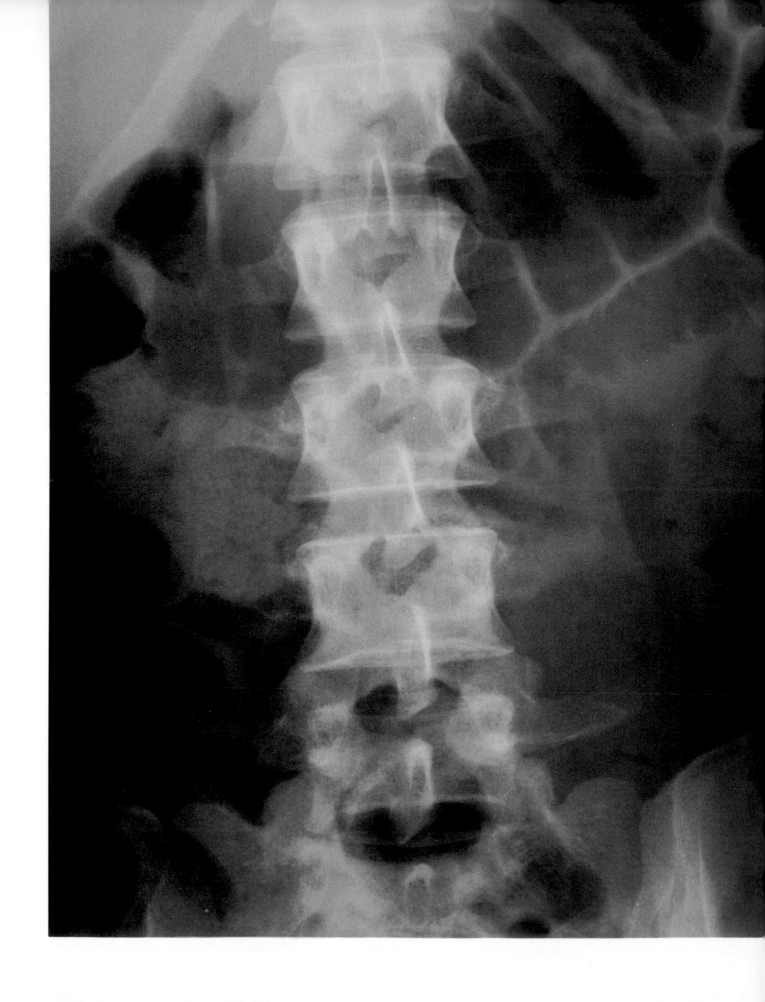

VIII. NEW VISION FROM TRADITIONAL TECHNIQUES

"Radiology is an apprenticeship, an old world apprenticeship"

A s I removed a huge pile of orange envelopes containing x-ray films from the seat of the only chair in his cluttered office, Dr. Harold Jacobson's phone rang. Jacobson, 76 years old and a statesman in radiology, still does a substantial day's work as Chairman Emeritus of the Department of Radiology at Montefiore Medical Center in the Bronx. He spoke with an equally talented radiologist who had called to confirm a diagnosis on a set of x-rays sent to Dr. Jacobson the previous day.

"Yes, it's mesenchymal chondrosarcoma. Do an excisional biopsy," advised Dr. Jacobson.

"That man is smart. If you are smart you ask for help. There is often honest disagreement by top level people in evaluating x-rays. Many people think a film has a definitive answer, only one answer. This is not true. Proper diagnosis comes from consultation. It's often a group effort."

Dr. Jacobson told me that even today with all the new technologies, 80% of the radiologist's work is in plain film radiography. There are over 130 million conventional diagnostic radiographic procedures

Plain radiograph of a lumbar spine to check for possible bone deterioration in a postmenopausal woman shows normal vertebrae and spinal disks. The film does indicate gas in the bowel and colon. Eighty percent of all radiological diagnoses are made using plain films.

performed each year in the United States alone. A billion films are exposed.

"A radiologist is only valuable if he brings a knowledge of pathology, physiology, anatomy, and biochemistry to his interpretation of a plain film. The public thinks we are black box men, that we fix radios. Often I hear a patient say 'when will my doctor look at the pictures?' They don't realize that a highly trained specialist with the experience gained by looking at tens of thousands of films is providing 'my doctor' with the needed information."

Traditionally, the radiologist has little patient contact: a technologist makes the exposures, and a radiologist in the quiet of a viewing room reads the film and records an evaluation. One radiologist told me he had never been taken to meet a patient whose life he had saved because of an exact diagnosis. In recent years, however, with the development of interventional radiology, mammography, and ultrasound, more radiologists are having direct patient contact.

Dr. Jacobson, who has spent his life teaching radiology, says it is today one of the most sought after specialties by medical school graduates, and 40% of the residents in the four-year programs are now women.

"They go into radiology because they know it is as exciting as hell. A radiologist is constantly dealing with challenges. You are 'Sherlock Holmes' trying to find the culprit by any means. There is the constant challenge and excitement of discovery. Radiologists love what they are doing. I never found anyone who wanted to leave radiology."

Since the 1970s, radiology has been further divided into subspecialties: neuro-, musculoskeletal, genitourinary, gastrointestinal, chest, and cardiovascular/interventional radiology. In addition, subspecialties have been created in computed tomography, magnetic resonance, nuclear medicine, radiation physics, radiation biology, and ultrasound.

Before passing written exams in radiology after three years of residency, and oral exams after four years of residency, the aspiring radiologist must be knowledgeable in all of the above. Learning the volume of information prompted by the explosive growth of new tools led Dr. Jacobson to remark to

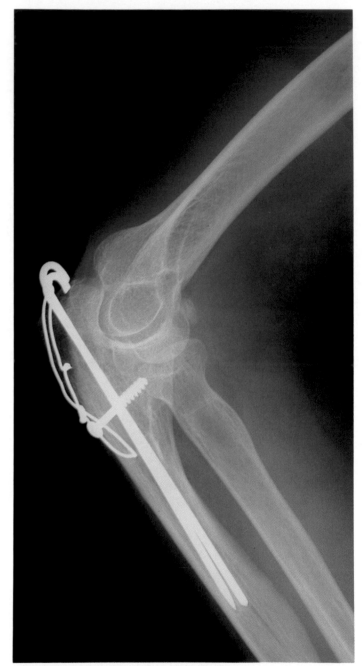

Lateral view of an elbow showing a fracture. A metal screw and two pins have been implanted into the ulna (the large bone of the forearm between the wrist and the elbow). Pins are inserted into the medullary cavity of the bone. This is a permanent implant. Radiography provides an easy method of postoperative evaluation.

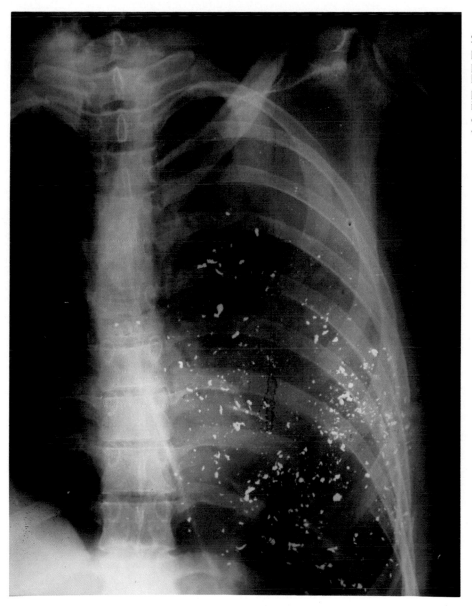

Steel shotgun pellets form an irregular pattern in the back of a crime victim. The pattern indicates that the fragments lie beneath the skin and have not penetrated the lung or vital organs. This is what doctors call a ``leave me alone case.'' The victim can carry the steel within him without danger to his health.

me: ''If I applied for a residency today, I'd get turned down.''

Plain film radiography consists of chest (40%), musculoskeletal (25%), abdominal (15%), and gastrointestinal (15%) studies. The remaining 5% covers specialized cases. In addition, a number of specifically designed techniques have been developed to facilitate radiographic diagnosis.

One technique, *tomography*, is used to prevent the overlay or overlap of information of one shadow upon another. This is common in conventional x-rays where the entire depth of a structure is being imaged. By using a focused beam, a moving x-ray tube synchronized to a moving film cassette, a single slice of information as little as 1 mm in depth can be viewed. All other information of lesser or greater depth is blurred by the movement of the x-ray tube and film. Exposure time is varied depending on the depth of the focused beam.

Where the radiologist is interested in a dynamic (moving) image as seen by the x-ray, *fluoroscopy* is used. Instead of a film, a phosphor plate is used as the imaging material. As the x rays hit the plate, a fluorescence occurs. Because the image is quite weak, electronic techniques are used to brighten the image a thousand-fold and a TV camera and computer monitor display the image in real time (in motion).

Another specialized technique, *myelography*, images the spinal cord and nerves. Normally, the cord and nerves are invisible on plain films, but by needle insertion of a radiopaque contrast material into the spine, a detailed look at the spinal cord and nerve system is possible. This technique, though now being replaced by magnetic resonance, has been used to view nerve roots and spinal disk protrusions, and spinal cord compression.

Other techniques include *venography* which involves injection of a contrast agent into the veins

Right hand of a banjo player; a leather half-glove in his palm.

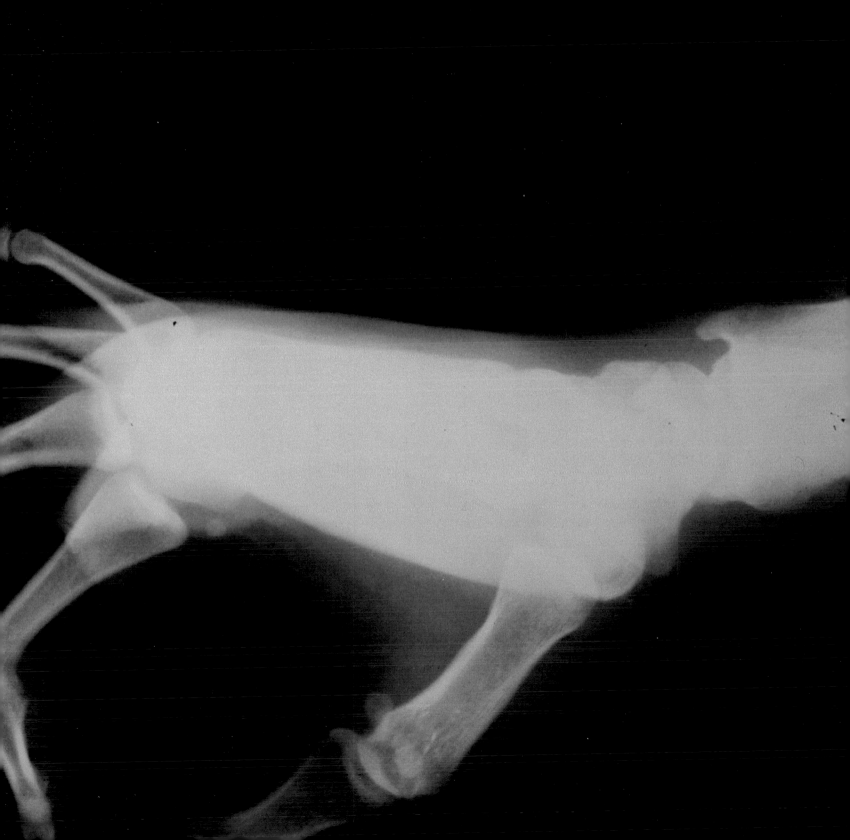

A radiographic view through a leather and canvas face mask used to immobilize a broken jaw in this auto accident patient. Only the round fasteners or rivets in the mask are visible. A few teeth remain in the mouth and the jaw is wired shut. X-ray films are a necessary tool used by reconstructive surgeons.

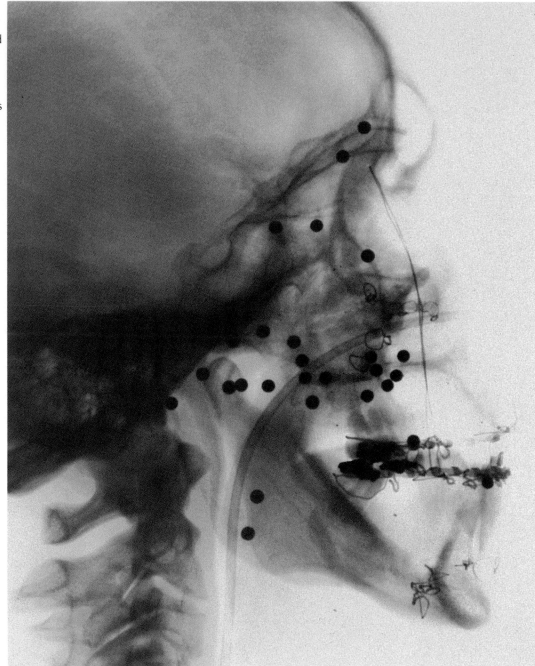

to determine venous abnormalities, *arteriography* to view the arteries, and *salpingography* a technique for viewing the uterus and fallopian tubes by the introduction of an opaque, water-soluble liquid.

In the past, the use of radiopaque contrast material has sometimes been avoided because of side effects in certain patients. More recently, nonionic agents have been developed that greatly reduce the number and frequency of side effects.

A unique application of cine-fluoroscopy can be found at the Johns Hopkins Swallowing Center in Baltimore, Maryland. Established in 1980, the center is devoted to patients with swallowing difficulties (dysphagia) and attracts patients from all over the world.

Headed by radiologists Drs. Martin Donner and Bronwyn Jones, it is a truly multi-disciplinary center. At the daily care conferences held each afternoon, medical experts from gastroenterology, otolaryngology, neurology, rehabilitation medicine, speech pathology, and radiology, convene to view films of patients with swallowing difficulties and to discuss the treatment approach.

The most common problems occur when liquid or food particles enter the trachea (the air passage to the lungs) instead of proceeding into the esophagus (the food passage to the stomach). In a normal breathing and swallowing sequence these functions are carefully regulated by coordinated action of muscles and nerves. Disease of the brain stem and cervical spine can also cause dysphagia as do strokes.

Swallowing activity is recorded at multiple pictures per second using cine-fluoroscopy, and the images are viewed on a TV monitor. The passage of food a distance of 5″ is recorded in 24 frames; each frame can be viewed separately.

On the day I attended the case conference, many patients' problems were discussed. One had swallowed lye; her esophagus was badly damaged and had to be repaired. Another suffered constant regurgitation of her food, and I was told it was caused by an inherited neuromuscular disease. In a third case, a heart patient had swallowed an encapsulated pill that had lodged in the esophagus, causing a lesion that was clearly visible on the monitor. He had lived on only liquid foods for over

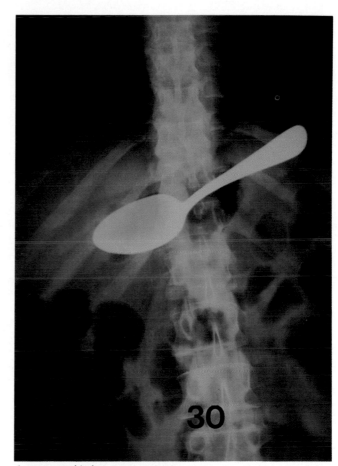

A common kitchen spoon can be seen in this patient's stomach. In time the spoon could pass through the entire GI tract but surgical removal was advised. This young adult suffered no pain and only slight discomfort after swallowing the spoon. Foreign objects are frequently swallowed by mental patients and persons under the influence of alcohol.

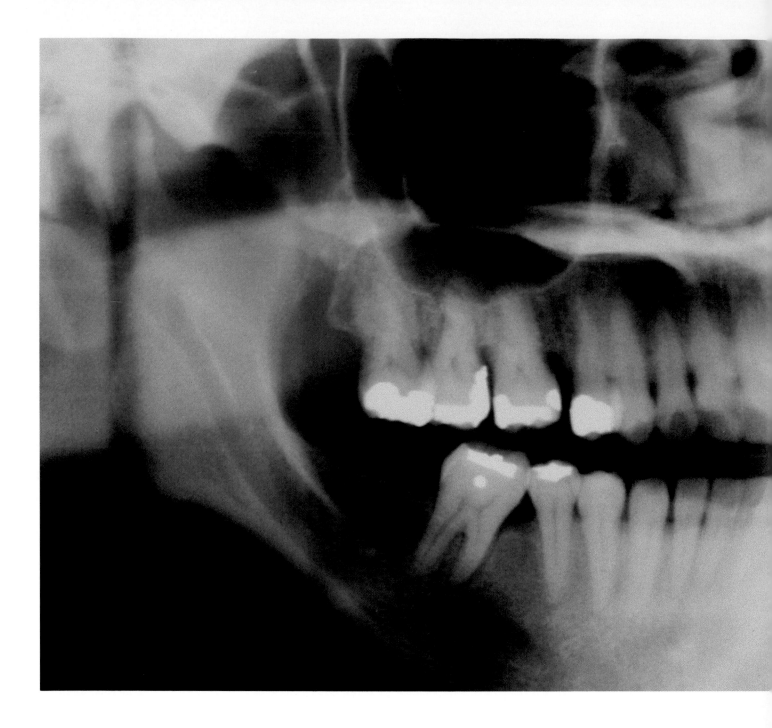

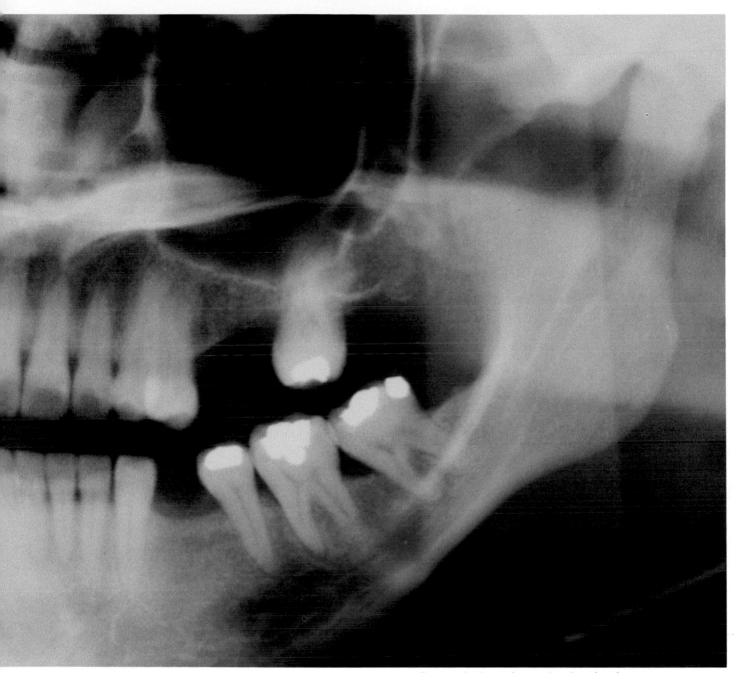

Panoramic view of an entire dental arch on a single film is a quick way to evaluate the mouth and gums of a dental patient. Note the missing teeth. The dentist's diagnosis was gingivitis of the lower jaw as well as resorption in the lower left gum. This middle-aged man suffered from chronic infection of the gums.

15 years due to the obstruction. His lesion has since been removed. In a follow-up visit to Johns Hopkins, he told the radiologist: "For the first time in 15 years I can eat an apple again."

Six million gastrointestinal tract studies are done each year. In the mid 70s, Dr. Igor Laufer at the University of Pennsylvania Medical Center in Philadelphia pioneered a new and important improvement in the contrast technique for imaging the stomach and intestinal tract.

The technique, originally developed for the colon in Sweden and the stomach in Japan, was refined by Dr. Laufer into a simplified procedure that could be used routinely. Now about 40% of all barium studies are done with the Laufer double-contrast technique.

Instead of the common method of introducing an opaque barium liquid into the gastrointestinal tract, Laufer has his patients swallow effervescent granules that produce gas. Then the barium is introduced. As the barium passes from the system some of it outlines the intestinal tract to define the folds of the structure. Films obtained by this method reveal much greater contour and detail than those obtained using barium mixtures alone.

Laufer has also perfected a method of barium and air instillation for colon imaging and a small bowel enema for studies of the middle regions of the gastrointestinal tract.

In the small bowel procedure, a small tube is passed through the mouth, into the stomach, through the duodenum, and into the small intestine. Barium is flushed into the system followed by methyl cellulose which distends the bowel and leaves a radiopaque coating on the lining of the small intestine. Laufer's contrast techniques have greatly improved image quality and are now used routinely.

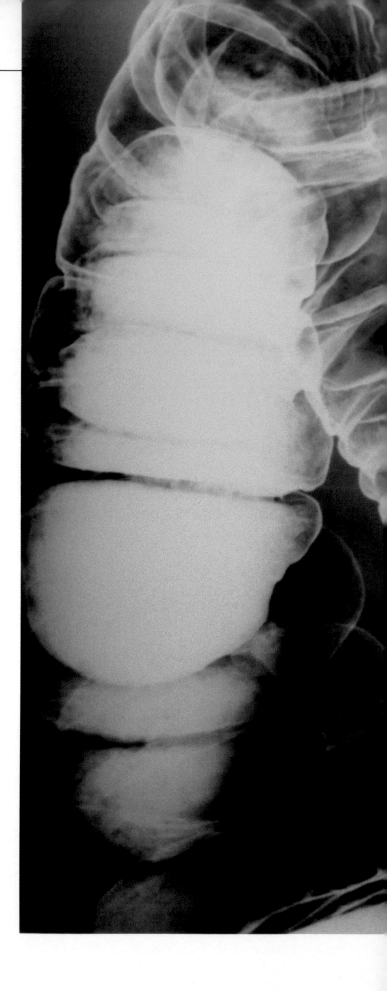

Almost 5' of the colon is seen in a graceful loop in this study using an air contrast barium enema. Descending, transverse, and ascending colon are all visible. A small black polyp appears in the bottom center of the film. This x-ray procedure is used to find polyps and carcinomas in older patients. Central lighter areas are where the barium solution has not been evacuated from the intestine.

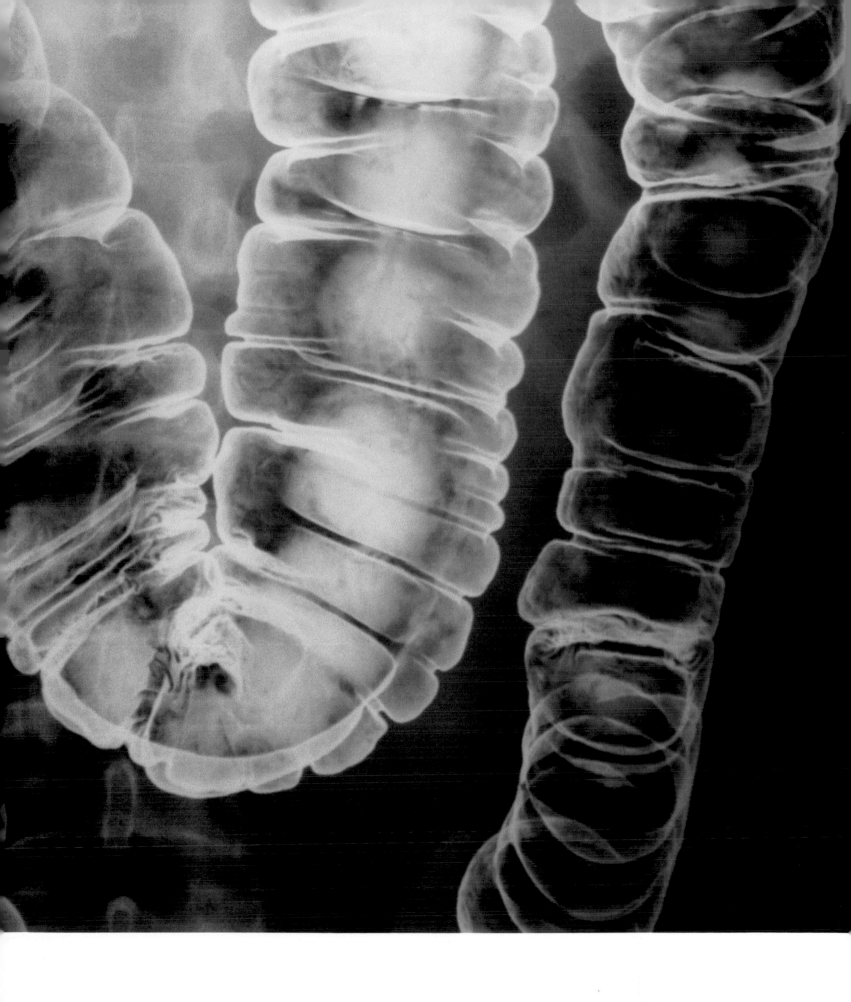

Pacemaker just under the skin in the chest wall pulses electrical energy to the heart from two wires that are attached to the right ventricle of the heart (lower right). Small, staple-like suture wires in the midline area indicate that this patient had previous bypass surgery. There is an enlargement of the left ventricle. The lungs are clear of infection in this 60-year-old man.

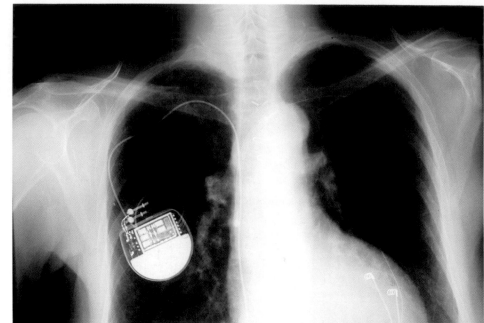

A thrombus (or blood clot) in the femoral artery between the pelvis and knee causes an interruption of blood supply to the lower leg. Note that collateral circulation has developed. Clots such as this often cause extreme leg pain. They are sometimes treated by catheterization using rotating drills and, more recently, lasers.

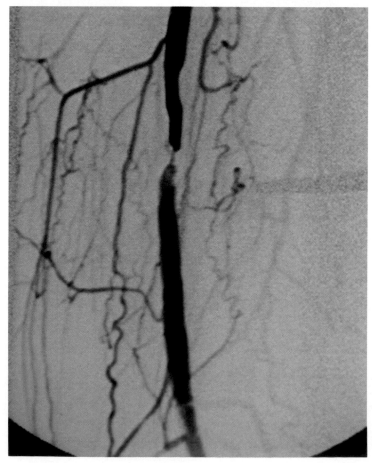

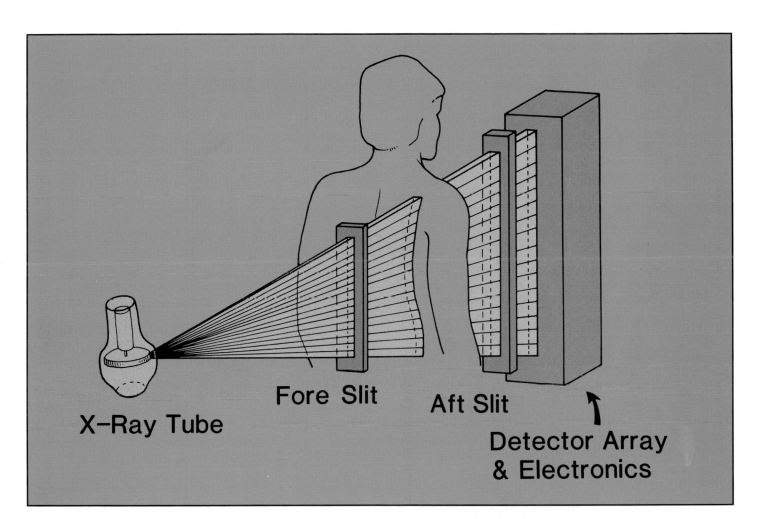

X-Ray Tube   **Fore Slit**   **Aft Slit**   **Detector Array & Electronics**

A growing trend in major teaching institutions of radiology in the United States is toward digital radiography. Film continues to be used as a permanent record, but images can now be formed electronically via scanned projection digital radiography.

In digital radiography the variations of signal produced by the x rays passing through the patient are translated into digital information by a convertor. The numbers, like the signal, vary according to the light and dark areas of the picture formed by the x rays. A series of coded numbers assigned to a picture area are converted into pixels or picture units. Each pixel varies in brightness. When reassembled by a computer, they form a whole image not unlike that of a radiograph. Picture units vary in size and govern the sharpness and definition of the final image.

Exciting progress in applying digital radiography

to chest imaging has been made by Robert G. Fraser, M.D. and Gary T. Barnes, Ph.D. at the University of Alabama at Birmingham. Here, digital chest studies using a unique apparatus have been ongoing since 1982. The apparatus consists of an x-ray tube, a fore-slit collimator between the x-ray tube and the patient, and an aft-slit collimator between the patient and the detector array. The x-ray fan beam passes through the 0.5 mm-fore slit collimator, traverses the patient, and then through the aft-slit collimator before striking the detector array of 1,024 photodiodes that are coupled to a gadolinium oxysulfide screen. The x-ray tube, collimators, and detector array move as a unit and scan the chest area of a patient in 4.5 seconds. Scatter radiation is almost absent in this digital technique. This is a major advantage over the conventional film-screen technique.

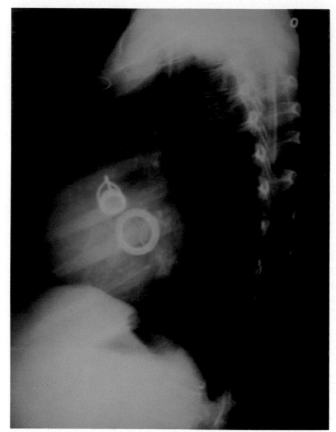

Correcting the malfunction of the two major heart valves, two implant valves are visible in this side view of a patient with an enlarged heart. The aortic valve is at the top of the heart; the mitral valve is below and to the rear of the aortic valve. The small suture loop (top left) indicates that a sternotomy (an operation through the sternum or breast bone) had been performed.

A second generation unit similar to the above involves the use of dual energy. Just as visible light has a variety of color values in its spectrum, x rays have a spectrum of energies. In dual-energy imaging, information from different photon energies is obtained with x-ray detectors that are sensitive to dual energy. A low atomic number phosphor/photodiode combination is followed by a high atomic number phosphor/photodiode combination to form a receptor sandwich. Low energy x-ray photons are absorbed in the low atomic number front section and high energy photons are absorbed in the high atomic number back section of the sandwich.

The low and high energy images are processed to obtain two images. One image displays only the bone structures; a second image displays only the soft tissue structures. This capability helps identify calcium in nodules in the lung and should make it possible to tell if they are benign or malignant. Theoretically, mineral content of bone, lung density, and inadequate blood supply could be quantified.

Drs. Fraser and Barnes feel that a digital unit with dual-energy capabilities can provide more information about the contents of the thorax (lung area) than is possible using conventional methods. The unit can demonstrate lung disease and reveals anatomic detail superior to plain radiography. By determining whether or not calcification is present, it can distinguish between benign and malignant nodules. Other abnormalities requiring fine spatial resolution can also be more readily observed.

A controversial but growing area of activity is the use of color in imaging. The advocates of color displays argue that the ability of the human eye is limited in discriminating very subtle changes in

Mass lesions in both lungs are shown in this digital film of a cancer patient. River-like threads in the lower left lung indicate chronic lung inflammation. Cancer had metastasized (spread) from the left to the right lung. Cure at this advanced stage is difficult.

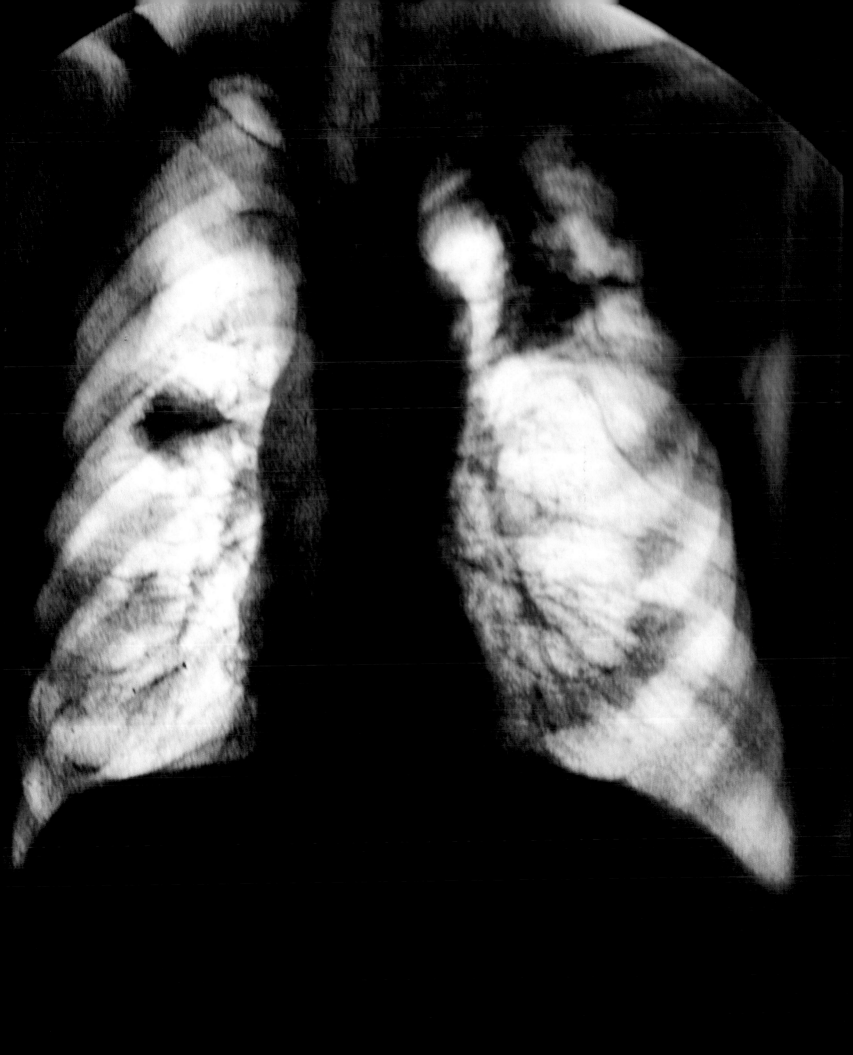

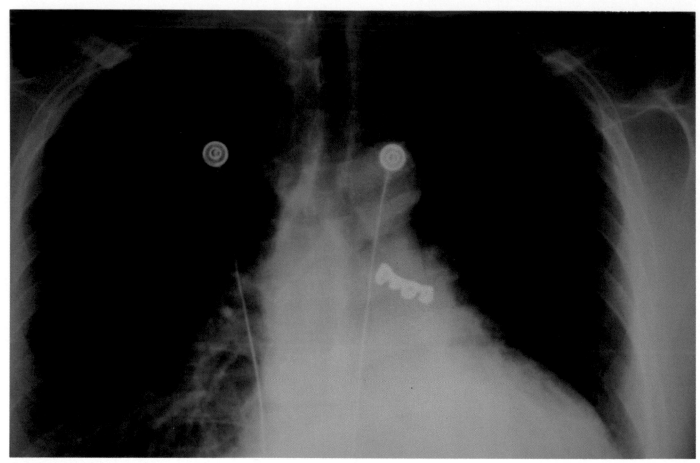

A denture lies in the bronchus leading to the lung. Electrodes indicate that the patient had an EKG just before x-ray. The denture must be surgically removed or it will lead to lung infection.

Frontal or anteroposterior (AP) view of the lumbar spine. Some of the disk cartilage shows osteophyte or bony outgrowth. Osteoporosis (deterioration of vertebrae) is evident in the lower area of the spine.

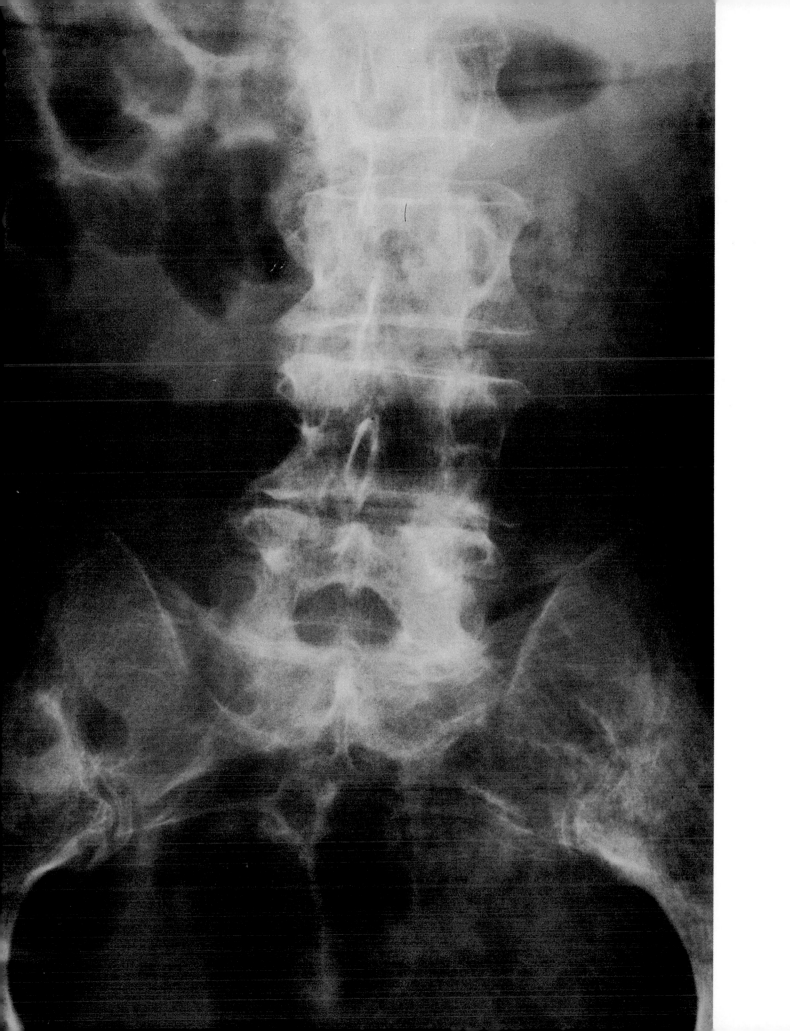

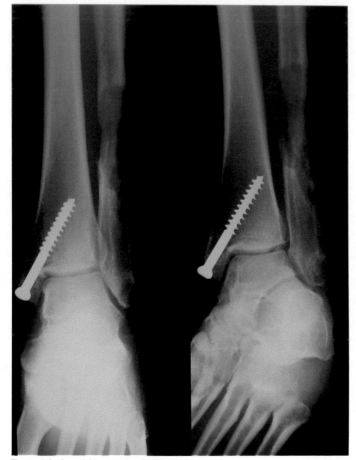

Two side-by-side views of an ankle fracture that has been repaired with a metal screw inserted into the tibia (larger bone in lower leg). The bone alongside the tibia (called the fibula) shows the presence of Paget's disease (shadow area, bottom right). The old fracture has healed nicely.

transmission of light through film of varying density. If we look at a gray scale with step wedges from black to white it is easy to see the blacks, the grays and the whites. It is very difficult, however, to see fine distinctions in shades of gray or near whites. Since medical imaging (CT, MR and all the rest) is based on evaluation of subtle changes in density, it is argued that any method that enhances the incremental changes would be valuable. The human eye differentiates only about 60 shades of gray (from white to black) but can differentiate over 250 color variants in a spectrum that runs from red to violet (ROYGBV). Hence, the human eye is far better at color perception than it is at black and white perception.

The Department of Defense has long used image enhancement in evaluating aerial pictures in camouflage detection, and more recently this equipment has been applied in medical imaging. Since electronic scanners are capable of ``seeing'' more than the eye can see, the original radiograph is scanned electronically and the image is digitized or turned into picture elements (pixels) as previously described. The new image is displayed on a TV monitor and each density is assigned a color. As an example, pure black can be changed to blue, pure white can be displayed as bright orange. Other colors can fill in the intermediate densities; assignment of color can be arbitrary or standardized.

Some of the images displayed in this book have been enhanced in this fashion to help the reader share in and appreciate the way radiologists see: the tumor, just a shadow, pops out in vivid red; the occlusion of the artery is easily seen; the yawning

X-ray of the legendary ``Elephant Man'' who was diagnosed as having neurofibromatosis (a genetic inherited disorder that affects one in 4,000 people). Note the massive buildup of fibroosseous tissue in the area of the brain. Tangled teeth are visible in the mouth. Small hook is where a ``trap door'' was cut into skull in postmortem autopsy, then hinged and latched.

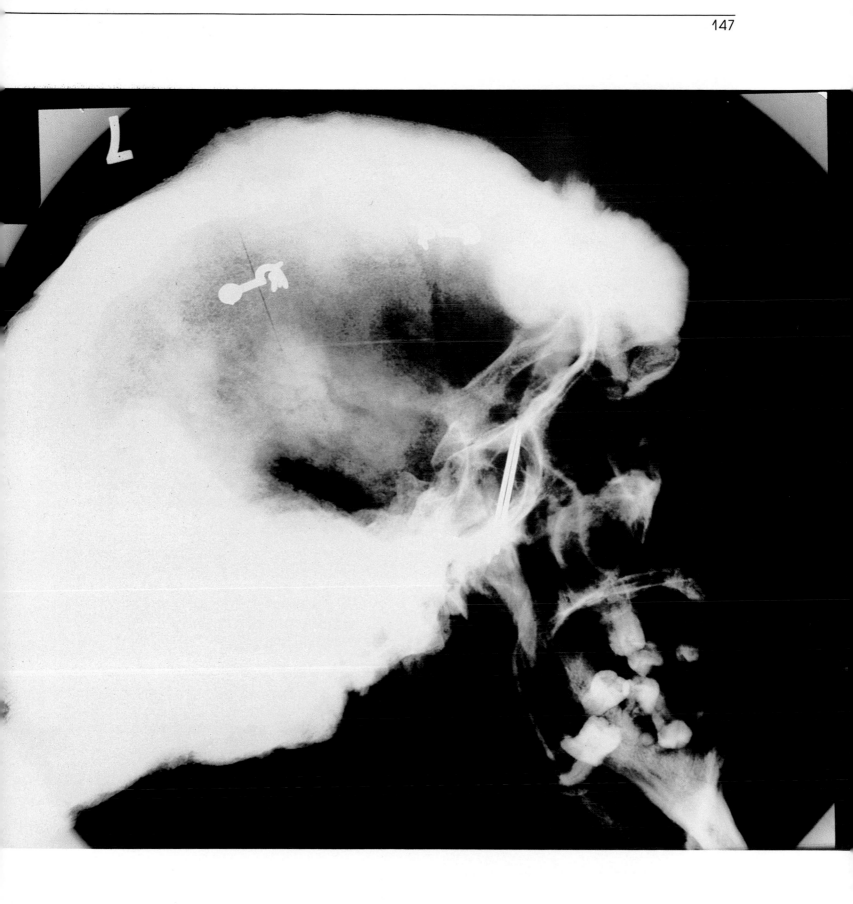

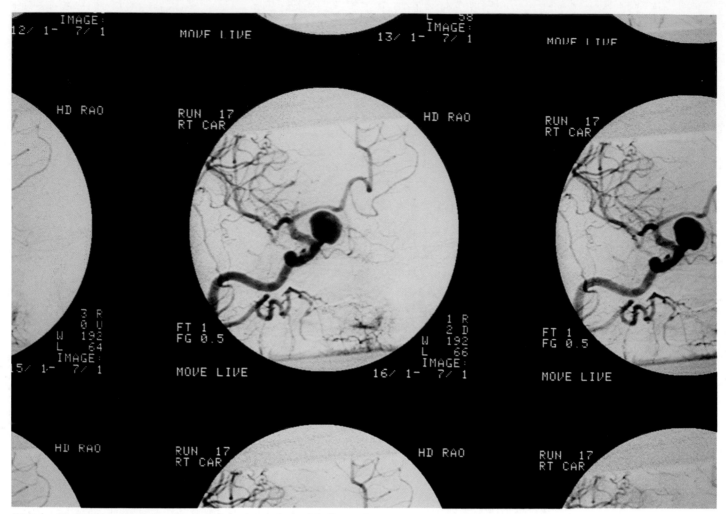

Digital subtraction angiogram of an aneurysm (a weakened, ballooned artery) in the basilar artery of the brain. This is a life-threatening event since it could lead to hemorrhage and sudden death. Embolization (a sealing procedure) is used to repair an aneurysm. Other surgical procedures also apply.

fetus comes alive. The argument against the use of color comes from professionals who know how terribly long it takes to develop the ability to read conventional radiographs. Only after studying thousands of images does the radiologist reach his or her professional peak.

With the introduction of color, a whole new discipline would be required. But with the advent of the computer and the imaging of physiologic function as well as anatomy, color is coming into its own. Doppler, Ultrasound, SPECT, PET, and some nuclear medicine studies are enhanced by color.

''Radiology is an apprenticeship, an old world apprenticeship,'' one distinguished radiologist told me. Radiologists are detectives, and their expertise comes from viewing thousands of films and formulating subtle comparisons. They learn by doing and their satisfaction comes from the excitement of discovery. Now, a technical revolution has taken place in their profession that has attracted the best and brightest from the medical schools into their residency programs. More progress has been made in the past 15 years in radiology than in all of its previous history. Even greater progress will be made in the next ten years.

The technical revolution in medicine has just begun. But no number of machines, scanners, lasers, catheters, digitizers or phosphor plates will replace the radiologist who must, with unique experience and keen visual perception, make an analysis and judgment that could mean life or death to the patient.

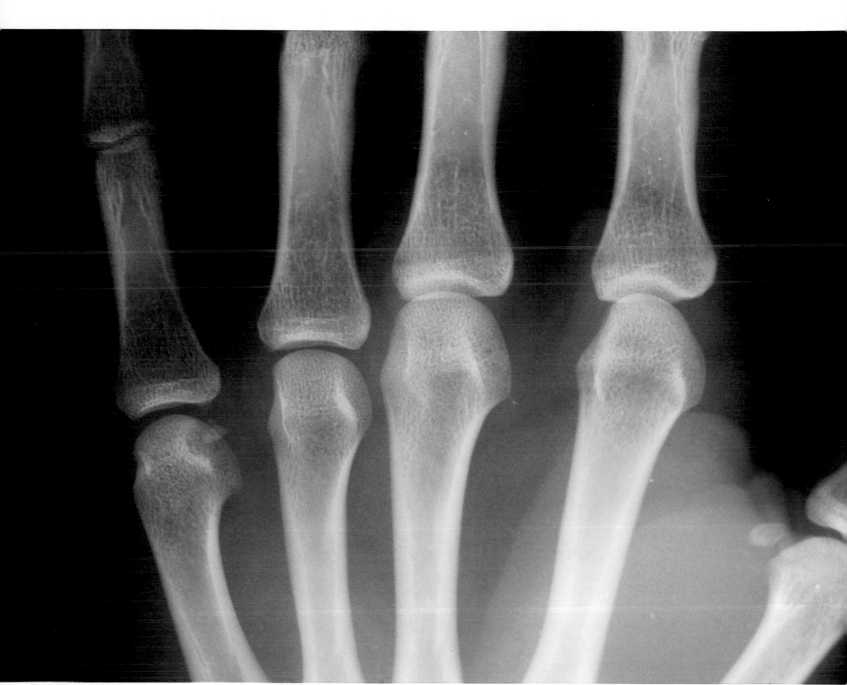

Fine detail of the fingers or metacarpophalangeal joints in the hand. Sesamoid bone tissue is seen in the tendons. This is a normal, healthy hand without any visible abnormality.

IX. WORK IN PROGRESS

*"Our ability to make pictures
is greater than our ability
to understand them,
and our ability to find problems
is greater than our ability
to solve them"*

The ability of a computer to digest
and display large volumes of
information, to sort it and make it
meaningful, is the basis of a new
science called "visualization."
Symbolic of the sorting process is
this data-packed view of a
terminal.

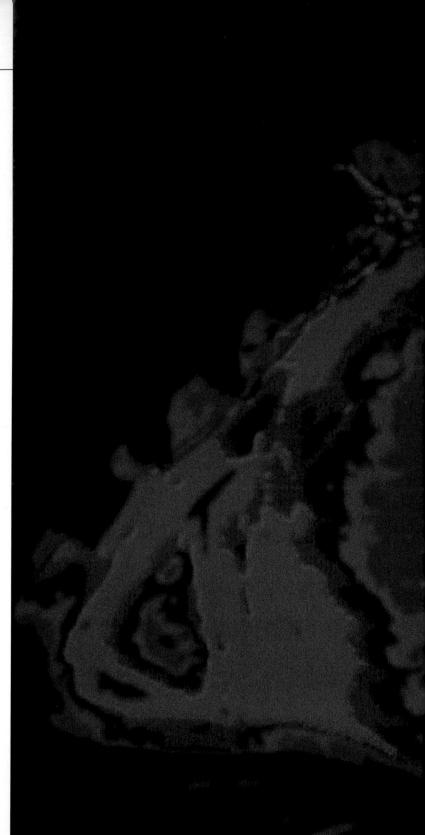

n estimated 50% of our brain function is devoted to processing visual information. More information of greater complexity can be conveyed by vision than by any other means. Herein lies the future and challenge of diagnostic radiology.

The computer has been central to the revolution in imaging. And as more and more information has been made available and the density of information grows exponentially, larger and faster computers have been developed to process this information. We have entered an era in which the computer has an ability to hear and see, and a new science—visualization—has emerged.

Computer visualization both interprets data and generates images from data; its goal is to provide new insight through visual methods. As the number of sources grows and the density of information increases (a super computer handles 10 billion floating point operations a second or 10 gigaflops) it is obvious that we will not be able to interpret this information in numerical form; the answer lies in the use of images. Visualization and computation will play a key role in diagnostic medicine as information is integrated from all of the modalities covered in this book.

The brain may be the best example of a complex organ where visualization can play a role in understanding its structure and function. The integration of all available data will be necessary to assure new and continued progress in brain research. Spatial distribution of neurons and brain mapping with computers handling 10 million instructions a second will be required. The output will be 3-D, high-definition images of portions of the brain delineating structures, and chemical and electromagnetic functions.

Visible light, that which we see with the human eye, is only a small part of the electromagnetic spectrum. Now other areas of that spectrum are being used to expand our vision. This image is a dramatic example of ``red-eye'' (the hemorrhaging of the tiny blood vessels of the eye) as viewed by infrared light. It is common in persons with a morning-after hangover.

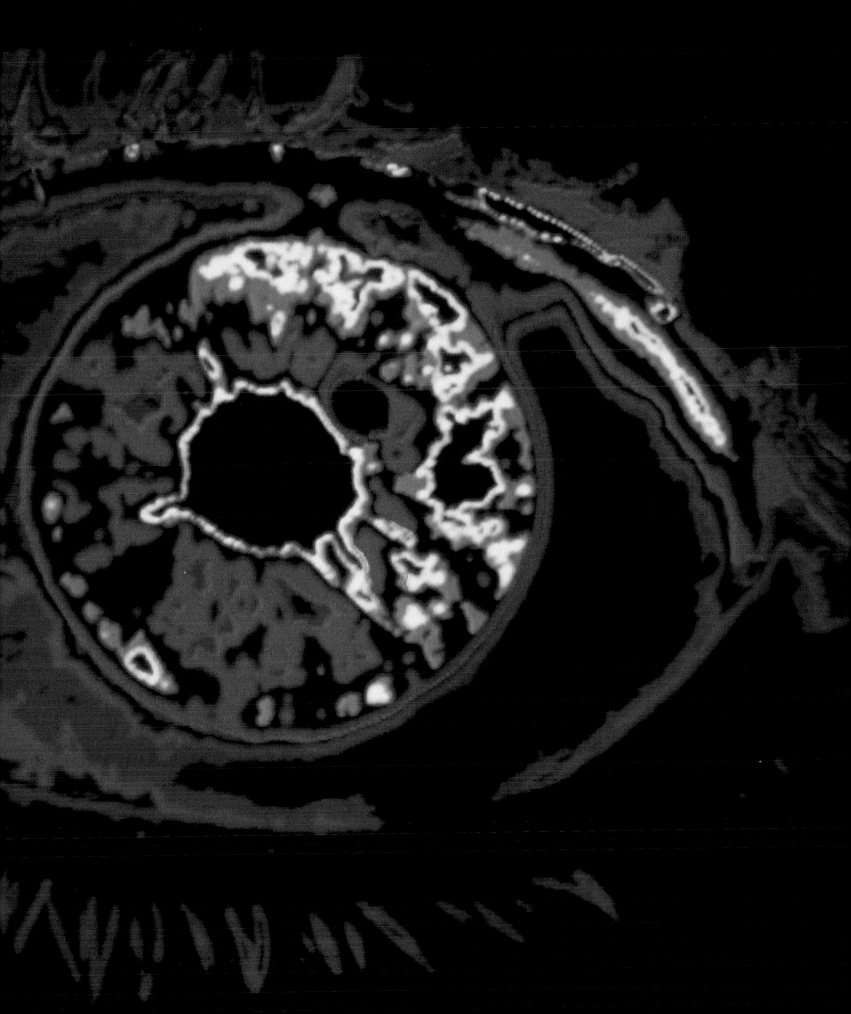

This three-dimensional image of a living skull was assembled from 64 CT scans to help plan reconstructive surgery. A portion of the skull, black central area, had been destroyed when the driver went through the windshield in a car accident. The surgeon, aided by this precise picture, fashioned an implant from living bone prior to surgery.

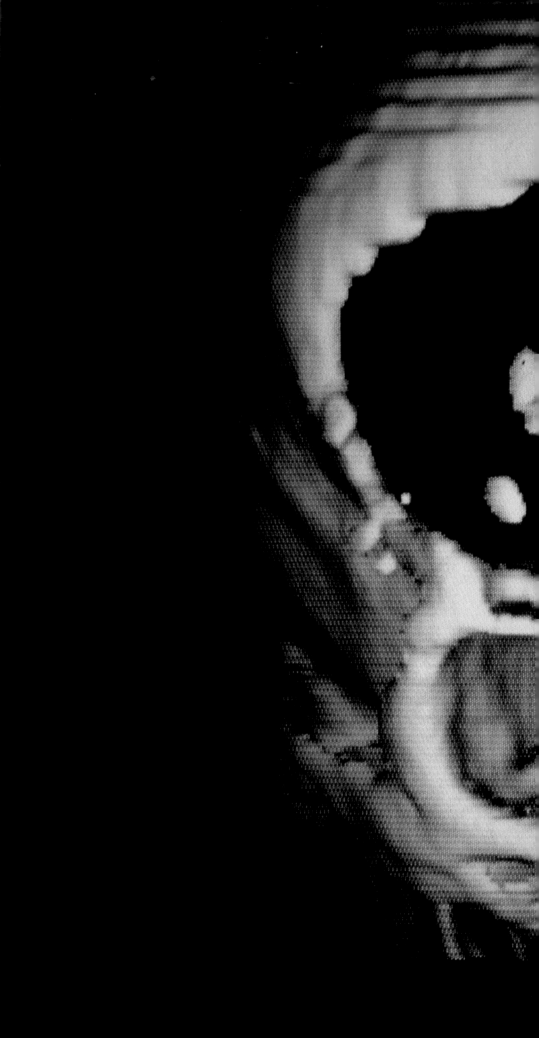

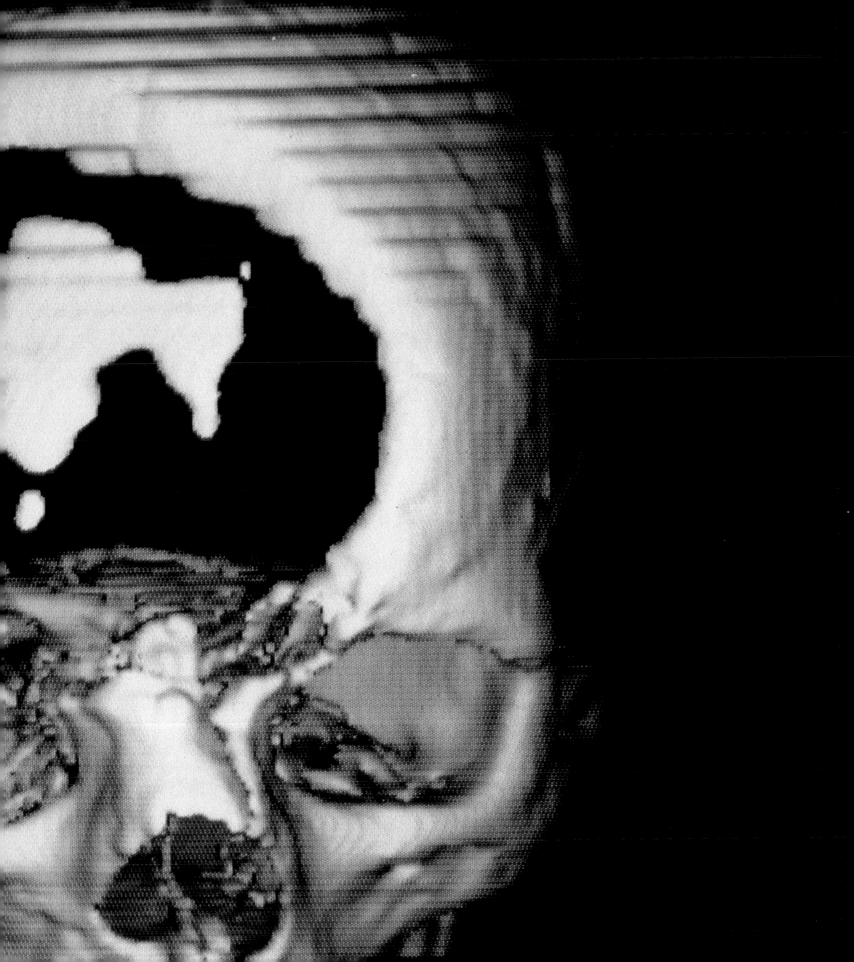

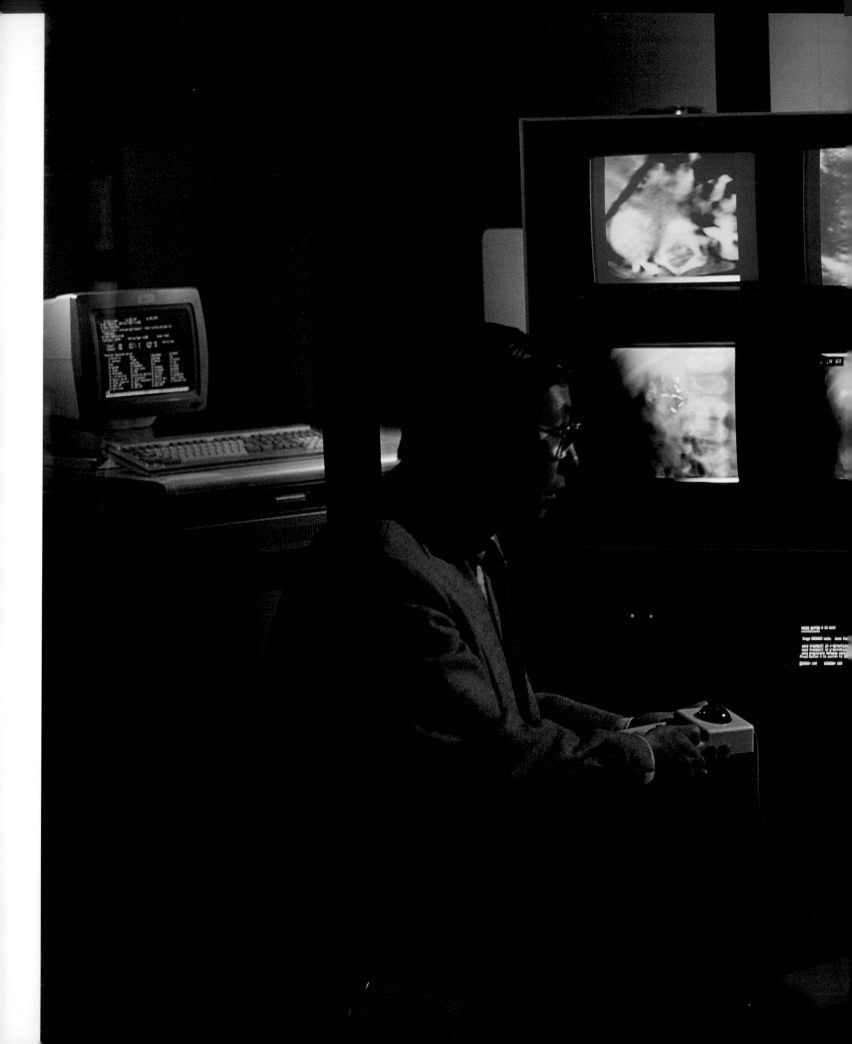

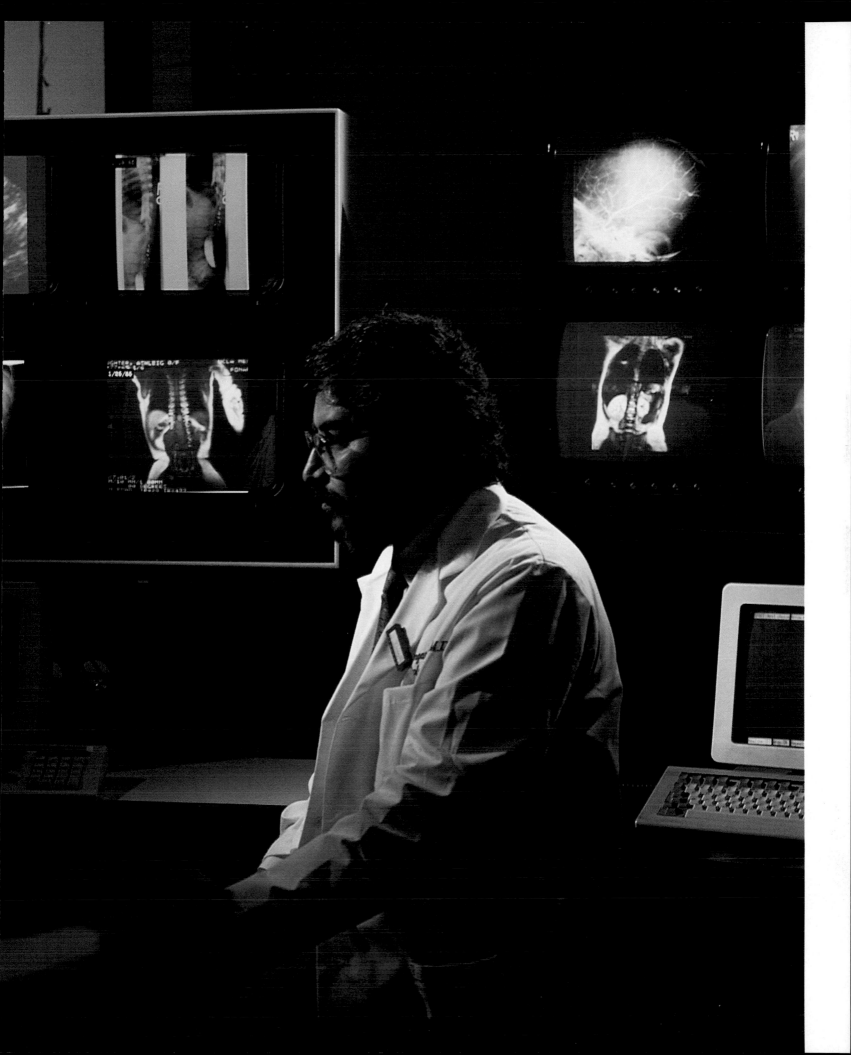

With the growth of computerized imaging over the past 15 years, an enormous amount of electronic information is being collected from every subspecialty of radiology. In addition to traditional radiographs which are an enormous storage problem in themselves (some hospitals have two or three people constantly shuttling back and forth to remote storage warehouses to retrieve films), medical institutions are now being bombarded with an ever-increasing amount of electronic data needing to be displayed, stored and quickly retrieved.

The answer to this problem also lies in computer processing. PACS, for digital Picture Archiving and Communications Systems, are now being developed at many major hospitals both in the United States and abroad (IMAC for Image Management and Communication System is also used).

A leading development center for PACS/IMAC is Georgetown University Hospital in Washington, DC. Under a $5 million United States Army grant to modernize the radiological services in military combat casualty care, Dr. Seong K. Mun has set up a pilot system to receive, digitize, file, and redisplay medical images. Ten workstations both inside the hospital and at a distant affiliated facility will be linked to a central data management system processor.

Simultaneously, radiologists and other physicians will have access to MR, CT, ultrasound, and plain film images displayed on computer monitors in the following departments: general radiology, nuclear medicine, radiation therapy, emergency room, intensive care unit, surgical suite, neuroradiology, ultrasound imaging, MR imaging, and finally the imaging center.

Dr. Mun's pioneering work has brought worldwide attention, and he has generously given his time to inquisitive visitors from Japan, Holland, Italy, Germany, and Sweden. His hope is that an international collaborative effort will promulgate standards that may one day permit medical image transmission worldwide (images have already been transmitted by satellite to Japan from the University of Pennsylvania Hospital in Philadelphia which also is active in PACS development).

Other PACS workstations are being developed at the University of California Center for Health Sciences, Los Angeles; Abbott-Northwestern Hospital, Minneapolis; Duke University Medical Center, Durham, North Carolina; Robert Wood Johnson University Hospital, New Brunswick, New Jersey; Baptist Bowman Gray Hospital, Winston-Salem, North Carolina; the University of Kansas Medical Center, Kansas City; and the University of Arizona Medical School in Tucson.

(Overleaf) Bringing together many views of a single patient, Dr. H. K. Huang of UCLA (left) shows Dr. Hooshang Kangarloo six images obtained using various scanning devices, each retrieved from a central computer bank. Among the first of its kind, this PACS system demonstrates the ongoing innovations that give ``new eyes'' to medicine.

A tumor of the nasopharynx, located by a CT scanner and centered in a cross mark, appears orange in this three-dimensional image. The imaging system is being tested and applied at New York City's Memorial Sloan-Kettering Cancer Center as a guide to aim radiation beams more accurately.

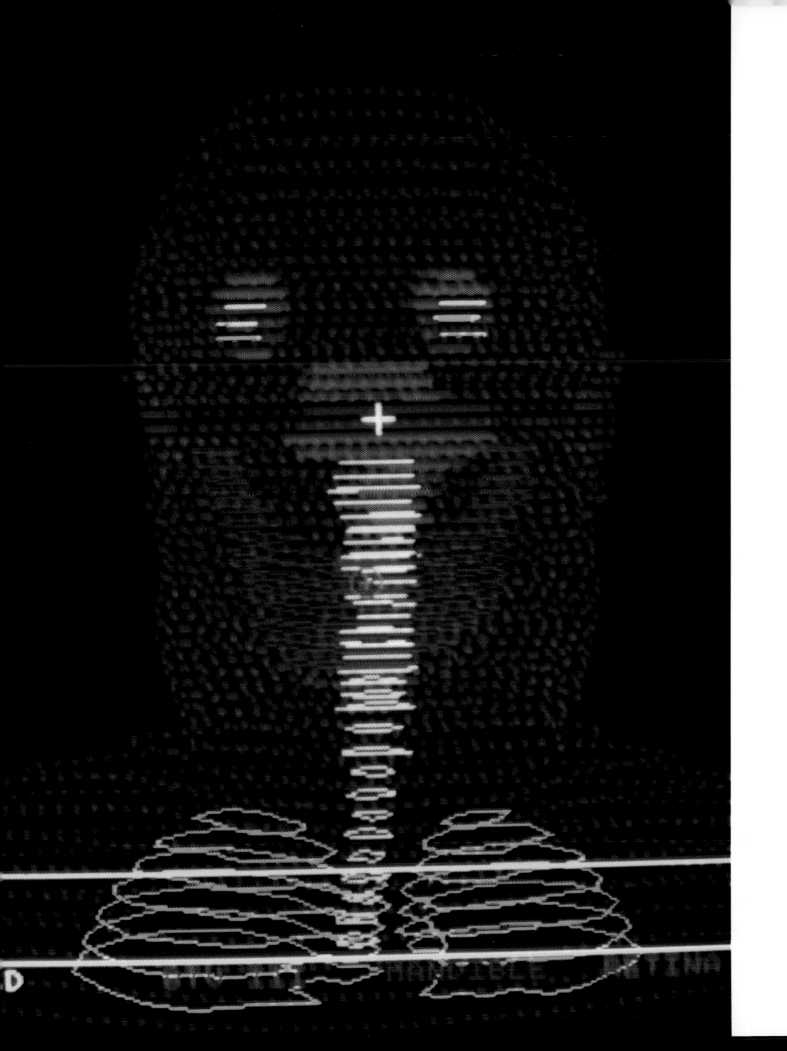

Still, much work needs to be done before these systems are in general use. Samuel J. Dwyer III, Ph.D. at the University of Kansas Medical Center has spent the last five years fostering the evolution of PACS. He points out seven obstacles that must be overcome. First, each imaging modality (CT, MR, ultrasound, etc.) has a different type of electronic signal input and standardization of data must be achieved. Second, the resolution of each modality varies and the current cost of high resolution computer monitors makes them too expensive for general use. Third, the best method of storing millions of images (magnetic or laser discs) must be determined, and new ways of compressing electronic data so that a minimum number of discs is required need to be found. Fourth, the readout of the stored material on either film or paper must be resolved (a scale of about 256 densities can be seen on film, only about 128 on paper). Fifth, the problem of tying the remote viewing stations together must be resolved—Should local phone lines be used? Should fiber optics combined with lasers be the transmitting method? Time, money, density, speed, and interference must be considered.

Sixth, a method of transmitting both visual and nonvisual information—in a coordinated way and at the same time—must be found. Images without patient information and case histories would be useless. Finally, the spatial resolution, contrast, and dynamic range of the images must be consistent and not electronically altered. Old images will need to be compared with new images, faded films with fresh films, films with high contrast must be as readable as low contrast films.

Dr. Paul Capp at the University of Arizona Medical School in Tucson believes all radiology departments must get started with developing the

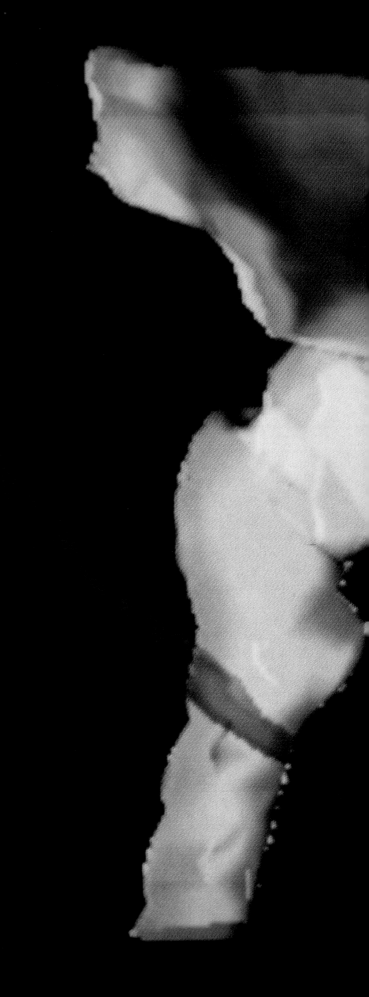

Area of radiation dosage glows red in this reconstructed CT view of a woman's pelvis. Brachytherapy (contact insertion of radioactive rods) was used in this patient (blue probes at bottom of frame).

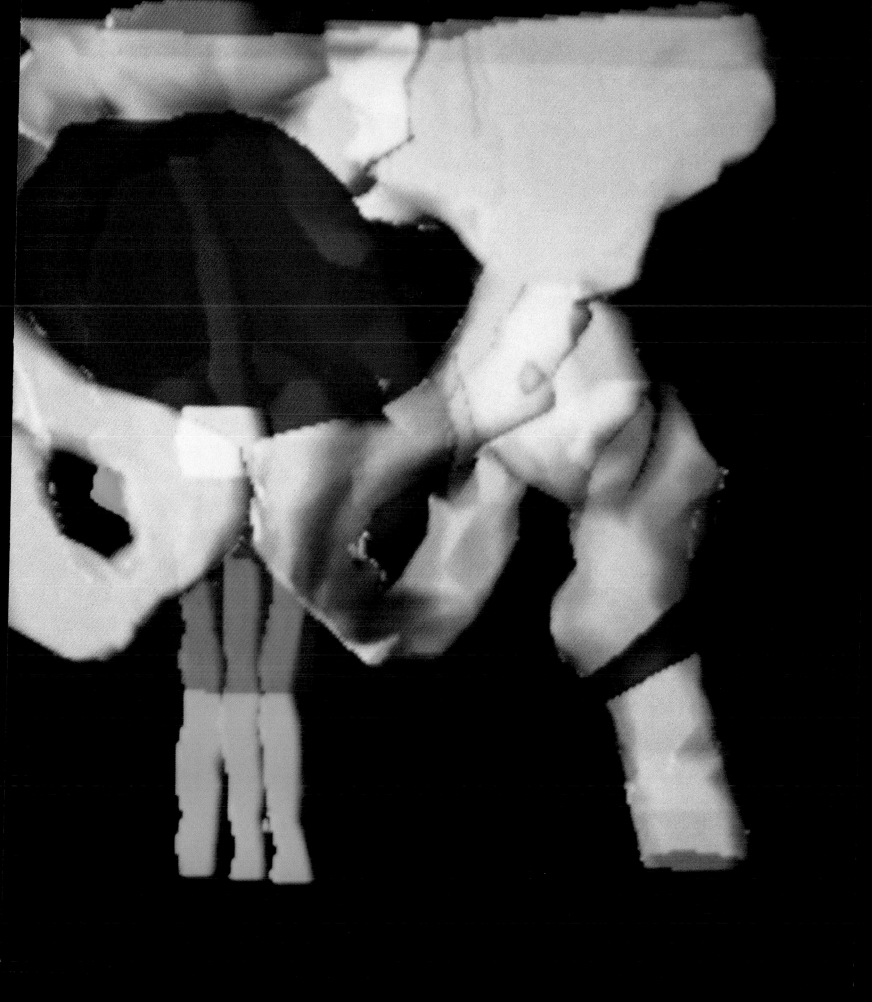

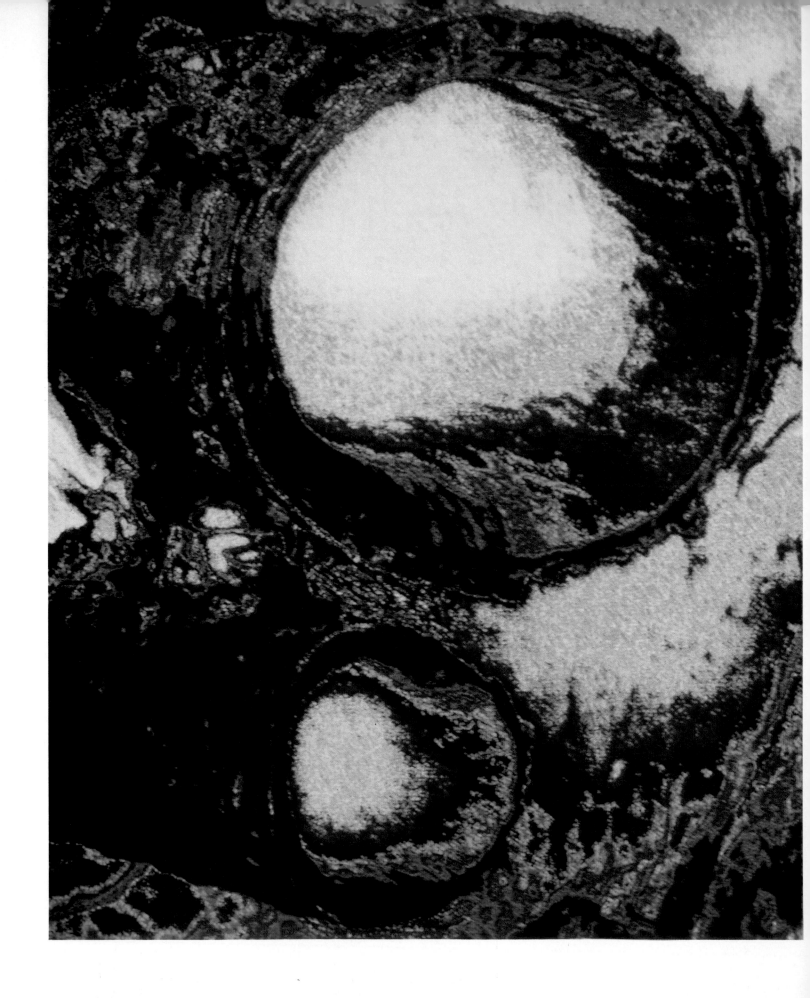

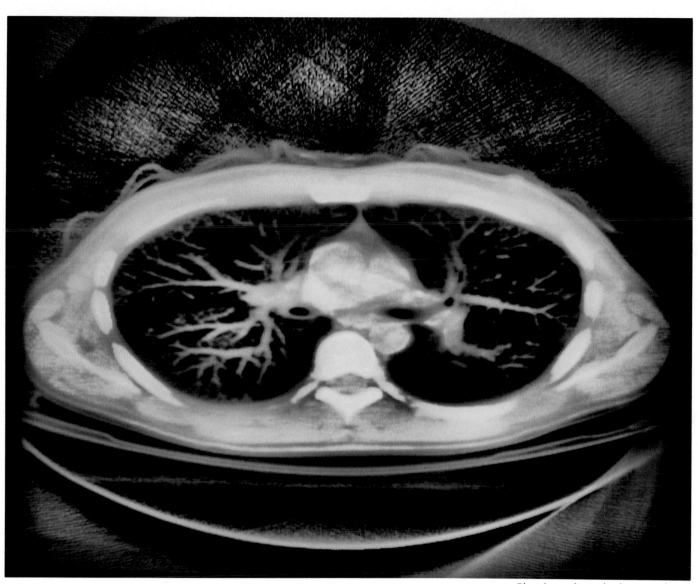

Blood supply to the lungs and a portion of the heart are seen in this axial CT scan of the chest that has been computer processed to sharpen detail and enhance contrast.

These arteries in the brain, pipes of living tissue three layers thick, were magnified 1800 times under a scanning electron microscope, then color enhanced. Arteries vary in size. The largest in the circulatory system is over a half inch in diameter.

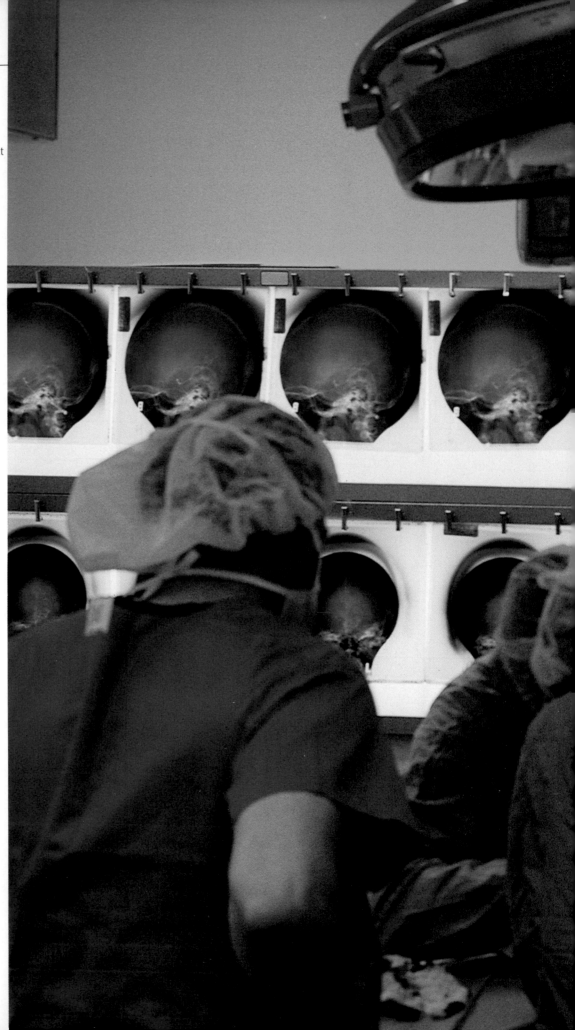

State-of-the-art operating room at University of Kansas Medical Center. Neurosurgeons here are installing a brain shunt to drain excess fluids.

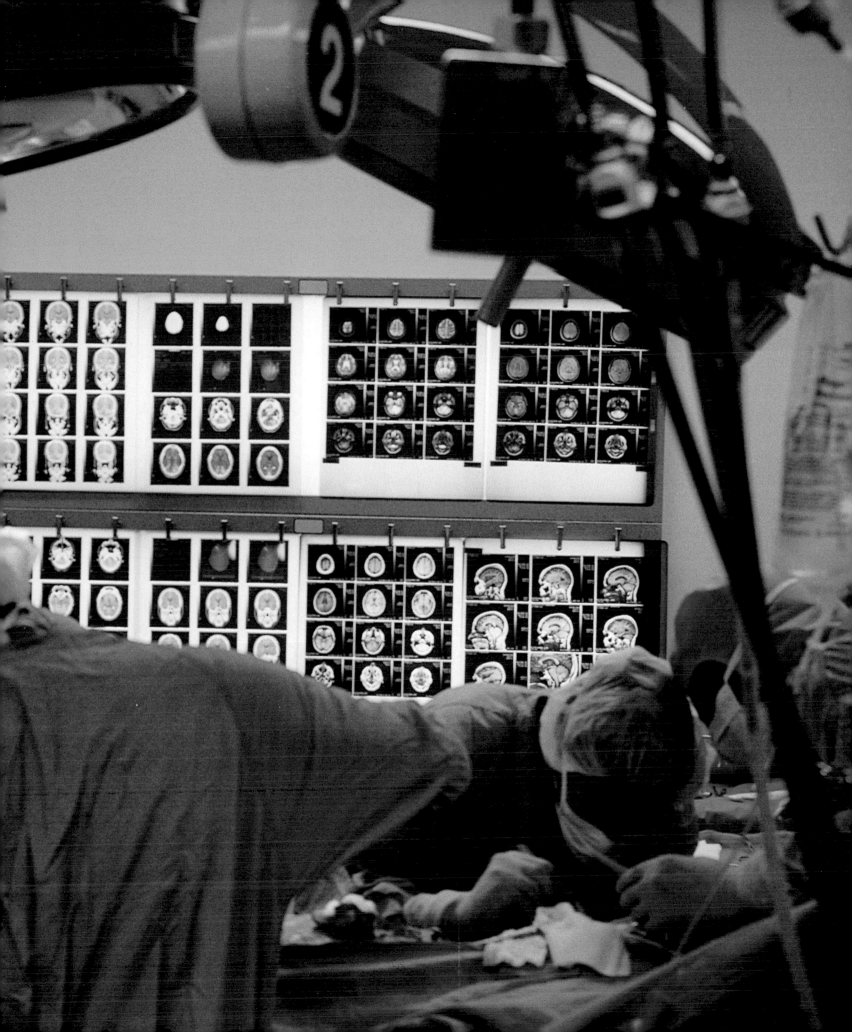

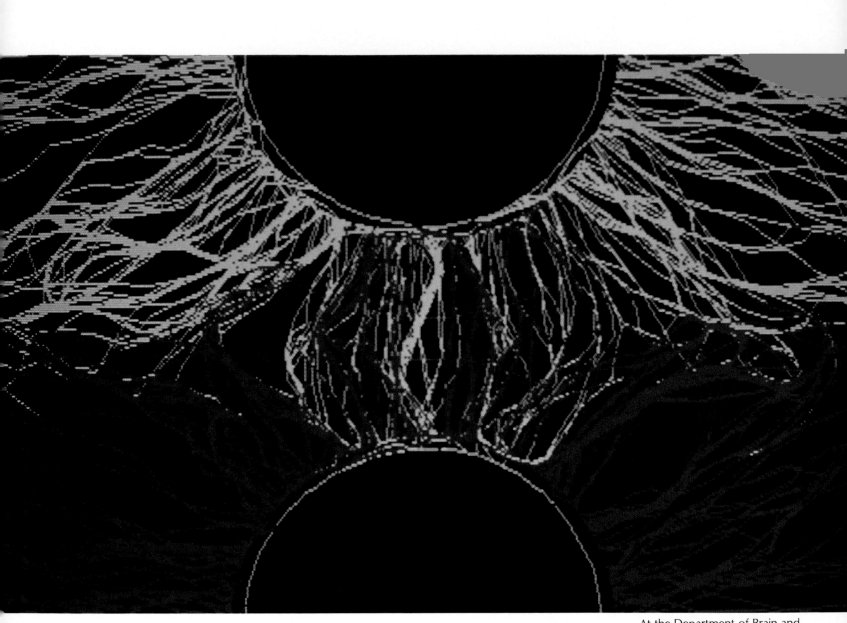

At the Department of Brain and Cognitive Sciences at MIT, brain cells grown as a culture send out nerve fibers that grow and interrelate. Based on advances in molecular biology and anatomical imaging, new insights into brain growth and structure are being realized.

all-electronic, all-digital department, and looks to the year 2000 when the all-electronic department will be a reality. He believes the 30-year time span between idea and application that has previously been the norm in medical science will be greatly reduced in the case of PACS.

What about the radiologists' reports that describe what they see on the images? Radiologists spend many hours each day dictating the diagnostic information they read from their films into tape recorders. This information is later transcribed into a report that is sent to the referring physician. Now, after years of research, continuous voice-to-computer-text display has been accomplished. The radiologist talks into a recorder that digitizes his voice information and instantly displays it in written form on a display terminal; it transforms voice to print. Now both words and pictures can be filed together in digital form for instant replay, anywhere, anytime.

In the chapters on plain film radiography and mammography, mention was made of screens put in contact with the film to greatly improve the definition of images.

In 1975, Dr. George Luckey invented a newer type of phosphor system, a storage phosphor system which, on exposure to x rays, traps electrons in the phosphor to store a latent image. To retrieve this image, a laser scanner of proper wavelength (usually in the red part of the spectrum) moves line by line over the phosphor plate which releases its stored energy to the laser. As it does, the laser is modulated and activates a photodetector. The information is digitized and displayed in visual form.

A dozen or so teaching hospitals around the country are experimenting with these new phosphor-laser systems. So far the results have been encouraging; the systems produce images of extremely high resolution, that have a dynamic range equal to that of film. Since the information is digital, it can be easily integrated into the PACS network in the all-electronic departments of radiology.

As the reader might expect, investigative work in diagnostic and interventional radiology is extremely costly. Department chairmen at major university hospitals spend a great deal of time in fund raising. The Federal Government remains the biggest source of funding. The National Science Foundation, the National Institutes of Health, and NASA having the largest resources. The National Institutes of Health as a part of its $6 billion budget has funded 24 centers for biomedical computing.

Several centers are studying "artificial intelligence"—making the computer resemble human intelligence rather than simulate it. It is a computational approach to decision making that has great application in medical research. Expert systems analyze the knowledge base and problem-solving techniques of hundreds of expert sources to come up with solutions.

Other centers are concentrating on computerized microscopy, molecular modeling, three-dimensional image displays, and very large scale integrated circuits.

The National Science Foundation has continued to fund six super computer centers where work in "visualization" continues.

The National Library of Medicine, a bureau of the National Institutes of Health has just made available, to professionals and non-professionals alike, a great medical resource largely unknown to the public.

A computer file of millions of medical books and journal articles, the Medline service is an index to biomedical literature of the entire world. This year it is providing a floppy disc with a program called Grateful-Med that permits anyone with a home computer to access the medical information stored in the center's computer bank.

Process of docking one molecule of the drug trimethoprim (for cancer treatment — white balls) into another molecule of dihydropholate reductase (red, blue, and green balls) is being examined in research at the Computer Science Dept. at the University of North Carolina in Chapel Hill. Piggy-backing of drug inhibitors is one example of an application of this molecular graphics project funded by the National Institutes of Health.

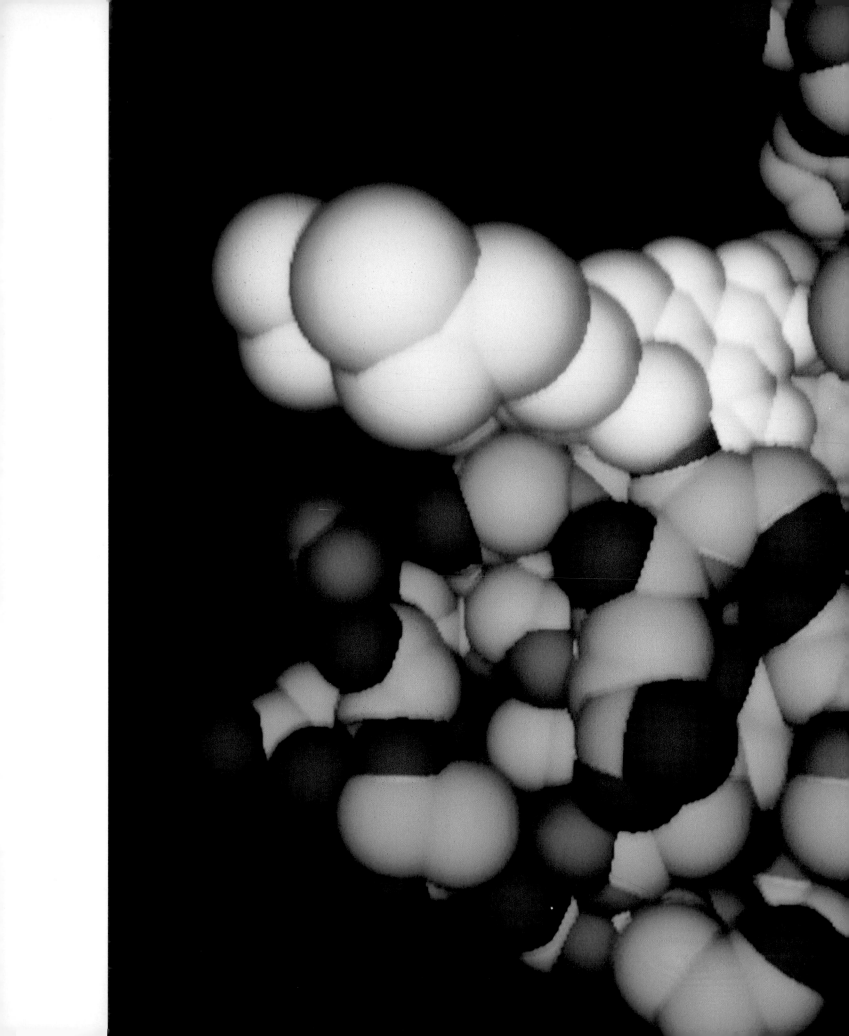

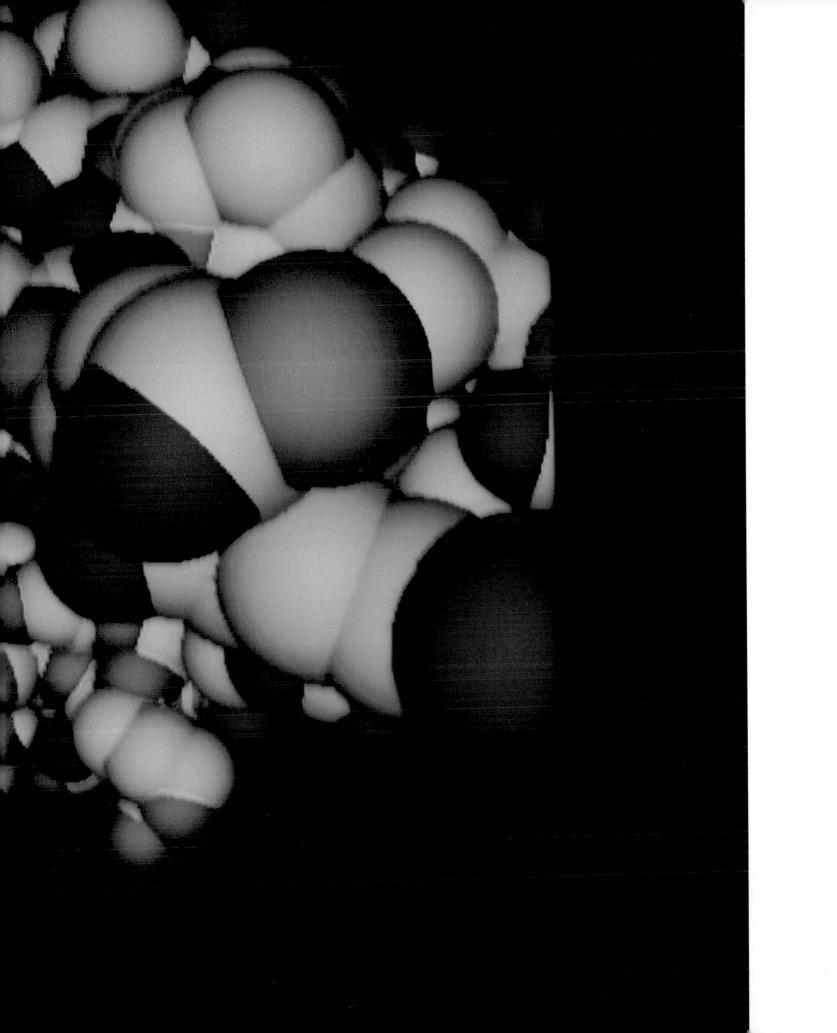

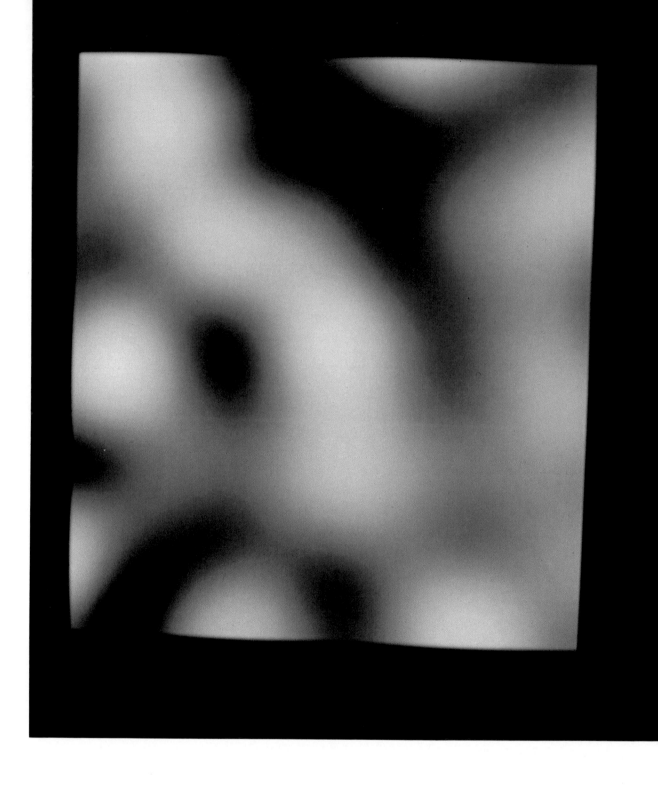

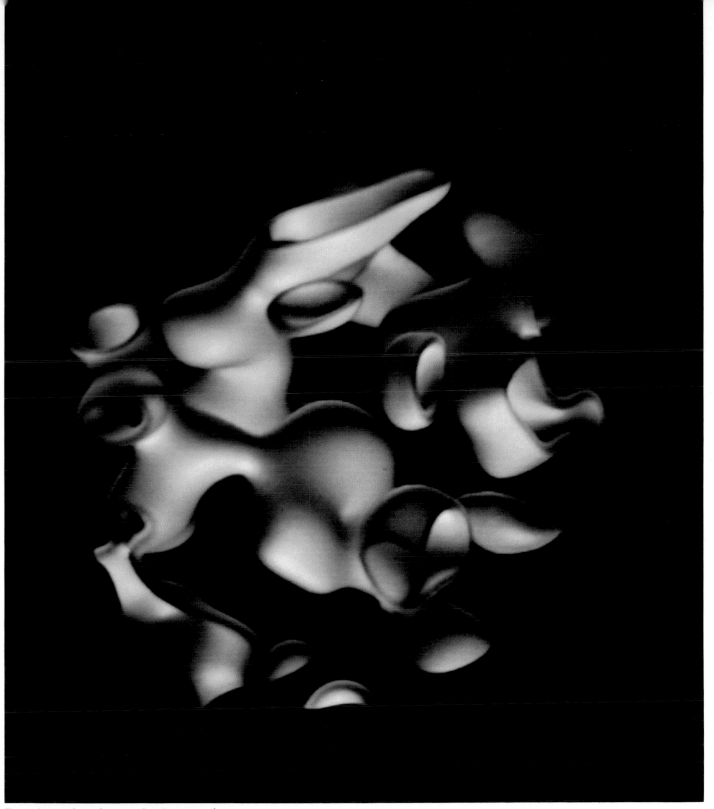

Two views of an electron density map of
cytochrome B-5, a protein molecule. Before
computer enhancement the slice is an indistinct
blob of gray (left); after enhancement (above)
distinct, 3-D electron density levels are clearly
defined. X-ray diffraction crystallography and
modern image processing techniques are
beginning to solve the hitherto unknowns.

Directed by Dr. Donald Lindberg, a staff of 540 updates information derived from 27,000 medical journals. Four million inquiries a year come from the United States as well as many overseas centers served by satellite (China, Kuwait, Egypt, England, Sweden, France, Canada, Switzerland, Italy, Japan, Australia, Mexico, Columbia, and Brazil).

For anyone with a home computer and a modem it provides a rich resource of medical information and is easily accessible to anyone, anywhere.

Three radiologists at the University of Arizona Hospital in Tucson are part of a formidable group of medical scientists brought together by Dr. Paul Capp, who heads the department of radiology. One, Dr. Tim Hunter, an associate professor of radiology, has recently published a remarkable book entitled *The Computer in Radiology* that outlines the computer revolution in imaging that is just beginning.

Another, Dr. Jim Woolfenden in nuclear medicine, has developed the miniaturized radiation detector probes described in Chapter IV.

A third investigator in Dr. Capp's department, Dr. Bill Dallas, has recently returned from the Philips Research Laboratory in Hamburg, West Germany to work on a project simply titled SQUID. SQUIDs (superconductive quantum interference devices) are tiny magnetometers that measure tiny biomagnetic fields. They are small superconductive rings with coils wrapped around them. The human body generates electrical energy and a current flows throughout the entire nervous system. Dr. Dallas' research involves imaging this flow. One application is in treatment planning for patients with epilepsy where distinct electrical abnormalities in certain brain centers have been carefully documented. SQUID and the investigation of the electrical functions of the body may one day form the basis of a whole new science.

Each year, in late November, the Radiological Society of North America holds its Annual Meeting and Scientific Assembly in Chicago. In addition to member radiologists, it attracts allied scientists, researchers, and interested observers from all over the world. This assembly fills the awesome and cavernous McCormick Place on the Lake with technical and scientific exhibits, and provides individual radiologists with an opportunity to share their latest findings with colleagues. A 556-page scientific program lists myriad activities including a subsection labeled "Works in Progress." By my count, there were 324 papers given under that title in 1987 covering the future of radiology. How can one hope to cover everything that's new in radiology in a volume of this kind?

In a very large sense the excitement has just begun. Few of us realize the tremendous technical revolution that computer technology is bringing to the field of medicine, and we are at the very beginning of that revolution.

I think the future of radiology lies in the tools being developed to provide new and better information, to display that information, and then to communicate it quickly and accurately to other users in the medical profession. Providing new and more accurate diagnostic information at less risk and cost is certainly the current direction of the profession. In addition, there is the challenge of coping with the great volume of information being produced so that it can be efficiently used and stored. The all-digital radiology (PACS) department with multi-image displays throughout the hospital and networks of transmission, storage, and retrieval systems will become a reality.

How often while preparing this book did I hear: "I couldn't have helped this patient ten years ago." Because of the computer and the new tools now being developed by radiologists and allied scientists, many lives will be saved in the years to come, and the quality of our lives will be improved.

Magnetic lines of force emanate from a solitary figure in this symbolic illustration. Man has progressed from cave painting to canvas to camera, and now to machine vision. Radiologists have been early to exploit this new vision which holds tremendous potential for the future. We are only at the beginning of a new revolution in imaging.

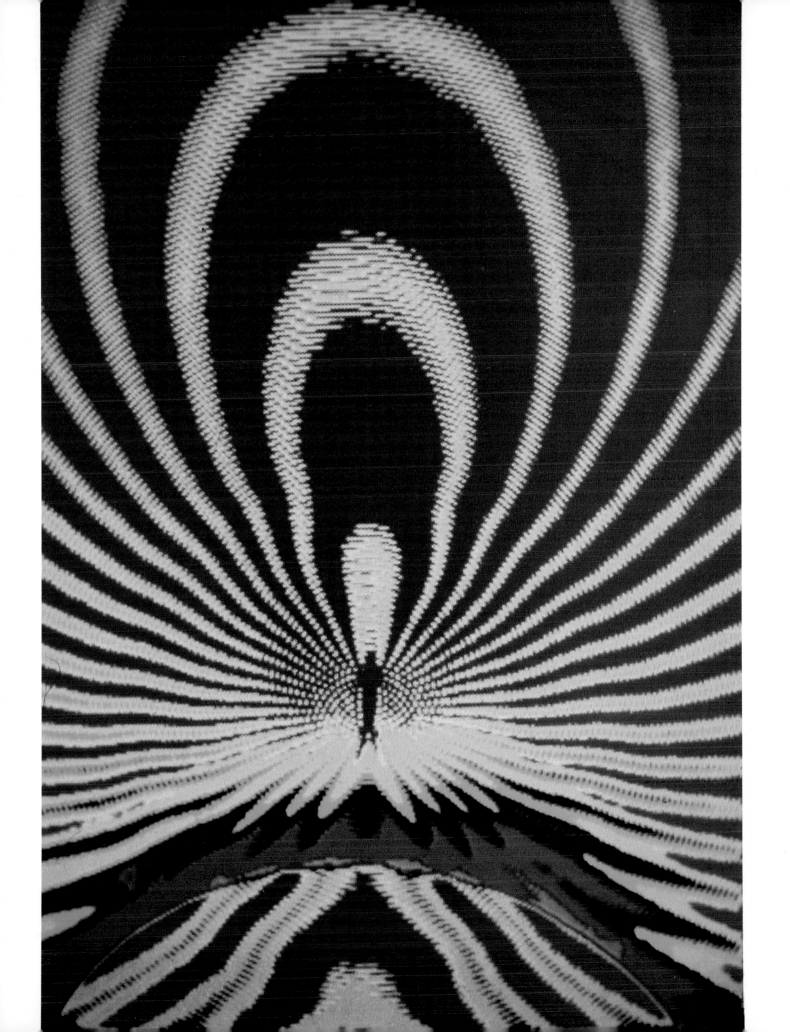

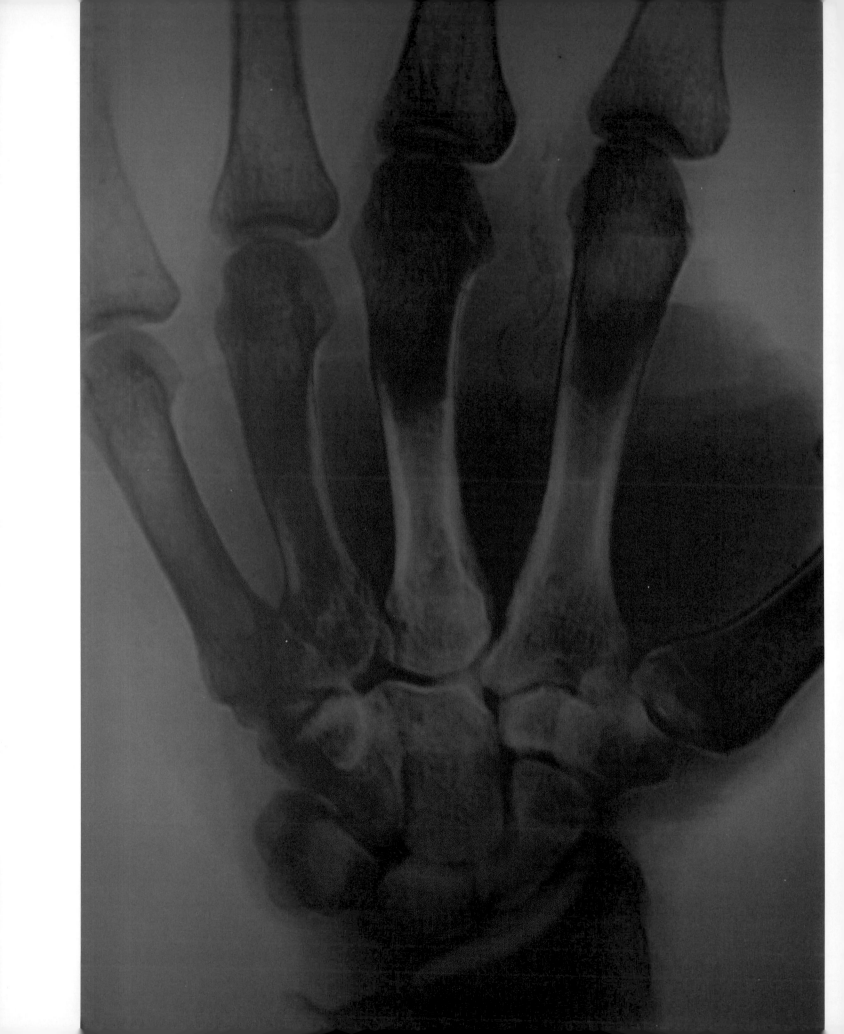

Acknowledgments

T he author wishes to thank the members of the Radiological Society of North America for their kindness and help without which this book would not have been possible.

Special thanks are due to O. Wayne Houser, M.D., who made many calls and wrote many letters of introduction to the scores of radiologists—overburdened with work and pressed for time—that I interviewed. Assisting him in these efforts and in review of the original manuscript were Robert E. Campbell, M.D., William J. Casarella, M.D., E. Robert Heitzman, M.D., James G. Kereiakes, Ph.D., Robert G. Parker, M.D., Edward V. Staab, M.D., and Donald A. Stewart.

Special thanks are also due to Arch W. Templeton, M.D., Samuel J. Dwyer III, Ph.D., Glendon G. Cox, M.D., and Larry T. Cook, Ph.D. of the University of Kansas Medical Center for their work both in preparing the original *National Geographic* manuscript and the preparation of the final book.

My copy editor, Valarie Stewart, revised, corrected and rewrote where necessary to assure technical accuracy and clarity.

The designer of the book, Anne Rhymer of Mack Publishing Company, put in many hours to marry words and pictures while maintaining an esthetic excellence of color and form and a simplicity of presentation.

Finally, thanks to my patient and long-suffering wife, Tania, who endured the past three years of hard work.

Picture Credits

Facing Title Page: Baby with bottle. MR scan courtesy Michael T. Modic, M.D., Case Western Reserve University Hospital, Cleveland, Ohio.

Facing Opener: Patient in scanner. Photo by Howard Sochurek. Courtesy J. Bruce Kneeland, M.D., Medical College of Wisconsin, Milwaukee.

Chapter I: Magnetic Resonance

Page 1:   MR scan of prostate courtesy Mallinckrodt Institute of Radiology, St. Louis, Missouri. Photo by Howard Sochurek.

Page 2:   Reflections in monitor courtesy James E. Youker, M.D., Medical College of Wisconsin, Milwaukee. Both photos by Howard Sochurek.

Page 5:   Painting by Davis Meltzer, © National Geographic Society.

Pages 6-7:   MR scan courtesy Mallinckrodt Institute of Radiology, St. Louis, Missouri. Photo by Howard Sochurek. © National Geographic Society.

Page 8:   MR scan courtesy J. Bruce Kneeland, M.D., Medical College of Wisconsin, Milwaukee.

Page 9:   MR scan courtesy Abbott Northwestern Hospital, Minneapolis, Minnesota. Photo by Howard Sochurek. © National Geographic Society.

Page 10:   MR scan of fetus courtesy University of Nottingham Hospital, England, Brian S. Worthington, M.D.

Page 11:   MR scan of heart courtesy University of Alabama Medical School, Birmingham, Gerald M. Pohost, M.D.

Page 12:   Photo by Howard Sochurek. © National Geographic Society.

Page 14:   MR scan of brain, St. Joseph's Hospital and Medical Center, Phoenix, Arizona. Photo by Howard Sochurek. © National Geographic Society.

Page 16:   MR scan of brain, St. Francis Hospital, Tulsa, Oklahoma. Photo by Howard Sochurek. © National Geographic Society.

Page 17:   Photo by Howard Sochurek.

Page 18:   Photo by Howard Sochurek.

Page 19:   (two) MR scans of brain, Vanderbilt University Medical Center, Nashville, Tennessee, Courtesy C. Leon Partain M.D., Ph.D.

Page 20:   (two) MR scans of the body, UCLA School of Medicine, courtesy Hooshang Kangarloo, M.D. Photos by Howard Sochurek. © National Geographic Society.

Page 21:   Photo by Howard Sochurek.

Page 23:   Photo by Howard Sochurek.

Chapter II: Computed Tomography

Page 24:   CT scan of brain courtesy Larry T. Cook, Ph.D., University of Kansas Medical Center, Kansas City. Photo by Howard Sochurek. © National Geographic Society.

Page 26:   CT scanner photo by Howard Sochurek.

Page 27:   Painting by Davis Meltzer. © National Geographic Society.

Page 28:   CT scan of spine courtesy Dimensional Medicine, Inc., Minnetonka, Minnesota. Photo by Howard Sochurek. © National Geographic Society.

Page 29:   CT scan of brain courtesy Larry T. Cook, Ph.D., University of Kansas Medical Center, Kansas City. Photo by Howard Sochurek.

Pages 30-31:   CT scan of pelvis courtesy Cemax, Inc., Santa Clara, California. Photo by Howard Sochurek. © National Geographic Society.

Page 32:   (top) Photo by Howard Sochurek. © National Geographic Society; (bottom) courtesy Steven T. Woolson, M.D.

Page 33:   Photo by Howard Sochurek. © National Geographic Society.

Pages 34–35: Courtesy of Larry T. Cook, Ph.D., University of Kansas Medical Center, Kansas City. Photo by Howard Sochurek.

Page 36: Courtesy Cemax, Inc., Santa Clara, California. David White, M.D.

Page 37: Photo by Howard Sochurek.

Page 38: Courtesy Elliot Fishman, M.D., Johns Hopkins Hospital, Baltimore, Maryland.

Page 39: Courtesy Patrick Cahill, Ph.D., New York Hospital, Cornell Medical Center, New York, NY. Photo by Howard Sochurek.

Pages 40–41: Courtesy Samuel J. Dwyer III, Ph.D., University of Kansas Medical Center, Kansas City.

Page 42: Courtesy J. Bruce Kneeland, M.D., Medical College of Wisconsin, Milwaukee.

Page 43: Courtesy Michael W. Vannier, M.D., Mallinckrodt Institute, Washington University School of Medicine, St. Louis, Missouri.

Page 51: Photo by Howard Sochurek. © National Geographic Society.

Page 52: Courtesy New York Hospital, Cornell Medical Center, New York, NY.

Page 53: Photo by Howard Sochurek at Long Island Imaging Center, New York.

Pages 54–55: Courtesy of Steven Horii, M.D., New York University Hospital, New York.

Page 56: Courtesy Rush-Presbyterian-St. Luke's Medical Center, Chicago, Illinois. Photo by Howard Sochurek. © National Geographic Society.

Page 57: Photo by Howard Sochurek.

Page 58: Courtesy Ochsner Clinic, New Orleans, Louisiana. Photo by Howard Sochurek. © National Geographic Society.

Page 59: Photo by Howard Sochurek at Ochsner Clinic, New Orleans, Louisiana.

Chapter III: Ultrasound

Page 44: Courtesy Rush-Presbyterian-St. Luke's Medical Center, Chicago, Illinois.

Page 45: Photo by Howard Sochurek.

Page 46: Courtesy Rush-Presbyterian-St. Luke's Medical Center, Chicago, Illinois.

Page 47: Painting by Davis Meltzer. © National Geographic Society.

Page 48: Courtesy New York Presbyterian Hospital and Medical Center.

Page 49: Photo by Howard Sochurek.

Page 50: (two) Courtesy Rush-Presbyterian-St. Luke's Medical Center, Chicago, Illinois. Photos by Howard Sochurek. © National Geographic Society.

Chapter IV: Nuclear Medicine

Page 60: Courtesy Brigham and Women's Hospital, Boston, Massachusetts.

Page 61: Photo by Howard Sochurek. © National Geographic Society.

Page 63: Painting by Davis Meltzer. © National Geographic Society.

Page 64: (two) Courtesy University of Texas Medical School, Houston, Texas. Photo by Howard Sochurek. © National Geographic Society.

Page 65: (two) Courtesy Ochsner Clinic, New Orleans, Louisiana.

Page 66: Courtesy Ochsner Clinic, New Orleans, Louisiana.

Page 67: Courtesy University of Kansas Medical Center, Kansas City.

Picture Credits

Page 68:   Courtesy UCLA School of Medicine. Photo by Howard Sochurek.

Page 69:   Photo by Howard Sochurek.

Pages 70-71:   Courtesy Brigham and Women's Hospital, Boston, Massachusetts. Photo by Howard Sochurek. © National Geographic Society.

Page 72:   Courtesy Harvard Medical School, Cambridge, Massachusetts. Photo by Howard Sochurek. © National Geographic Society.

Page 73:   Photo by Howard Sochurek taken at University of Kansas Medical Center, Kansas City.

Page 75:   Courtesy Emory University School of Medicine, Atlanta, Georgia.

Pages 84-85:   Photos by Howard Sochurek taken at University of Arkansas Barton Research Center, Little Rock, and Cincinnati Children's Hospital, Ohio.

Pages 86-87:   Photo by Howard Sochurek. © National Geographic Society.

Page 88:   Photo by Howard Sochurek.

Page 89:   Computer generated image courtesy of Megavision, Inc., Santa Barbara, California.

Page 90:   Photo by Howard Sochurek at NYU Medical Center.

Pages 91, 93:   Photos by Howard Sochurek taken at the University of Arizona Hospital and Medical School, Tucson.

Chapter V: Interventional Radiology

Page 76:   Courtesy University of Kansas Medical Center, Kansas City. Photo by Howard Sochurek. © National Geographic Society.

Page 77:   Photo by Howard Sochurek. © National Geographic Society.

Page 78:   Photo by Howard Sochurek at NYU Medical Center.

Page 79:   Painting by Davis Meltzer. © National Geographic Society.

Page 80:   (two) Courtesy East Jefferson General Hospital, New Orleans, Louisiana. Photos by Howard Sochurek. © National Geographic Society.

Page 81:   Photo by Howard Sochurek. © National Geographic Society.

Page 82:   Photo by Howard Sochurek.

Page 83:   Courtesy Fischer Imaging Corporation, Denver, Colorado. Photo by Howard Sochurek. © National Geographic Society.

Chapter VI: Radiation Therapy

Page 94:   Photo by Howard Sochurek taken at Neutron Therapy Facility at UCLA.

Page 95:   Photo by Howard Sochurek taken at Wadsworth VA Hospital, Los Angeles, California.

Pages 96, 97:   Photo by Howard Sochurek taken at Wadsworth VA Hospital, Los Angeles, California.

Pages 99, 100:   Courtesy Memorial Sloan-Kettering Cancer Center, New York. Photo by Howard Sochurek. © National Geographic Society.

Page 102:   (three) Courtesy of Stephen M. Pizer, Ph.D., Department of Computer Science, University of North Carolina at Chapel Hill.

Page 103:   Courtesy Marc R. Sontag, Ph.D., University of Pennsylvania School of Medicine, Philadelphia.

Page 104:   Courtesy of Julian Rosenman, M.D., and George W. Sherouse, M.S., North Carolina Memorial Hospital, Chapel Hill.

Pages 105-109:   Photos by Howard Sochurek.

Chapter VII: Mammography

Page 111:   Courtesy of West Side Radiology Associates, P.C., affiliated with St. Lukes-Roosevelt Hospital Center, New York.

Page 112:   Courtesy National Institutes of Health, Bethesda, Maryland.

Page 113:   Courtesy Wende Logan, M.D., Rochester, New York.

Page 114:   Photo by Howard Sochurek at West Side Radiology Associates, P.C., New York.

Page 115:   Courtesy Memorial Sloan-Kettering Cancer Center, New York.

Page 116:   Courtesy George Crile, Jr., M.D., Cleveland Clinic, Cleveland, Ohio.

Pages 118-119, 121:   Photo by Howard Sochurek.

Pages 122, 123:   Courtesy University of Kansas Medical Center, Kansas City.

Pages 124, 125:   Courtesy University of North Carolina, Department of Computer Science, Chapel Hill.

Page 127:   Courtesy Megavision Inc., Santa Barbara, California.

Chapter VIII: New Vision From Traditional Techniques

Pages 128, 130-134, 136-140 (bottom), 143, 145, 146, 148, 149:   Courtesy Eastman Kodak Company, Health Sciences Division, Rochester, New York, (permanent collection).

Page 135:   Courtesy of Benjamin Felson, M.D., (permanent collection) University Hospital, Cincinnati, Ohio.

Page 140:   Courtesy Sanford A. Rubin, M.D., collection at University of Texas Medical Branch, Galveston.

Page 141:   Courtesy of Robert G. Fraser, M.D., University of Alabama in Birmingham.

Pages 142, 144:   Courtesy of Sanford A. Rubin, M.D., University of Texas Medical Branch, Galveston.

Page 147:   Courtesy Benjamin Felson, M.D., University Hospital, Cincinnati, Ohio.

Chapter IX: Works in Progress

Pages 150, 151:   Photo by Howard Sochurek using Megavision (Santa Barbara, California) processing.

Pages 152, 153:   Photo by Howard Sochurek.

Pages 154, 155:   Courtesy Cemax, Inc., Santa Clara, California.

Pages 156, 157:   Photo by Howard Sochurek taken at UCLA Medical Center, Division of Medical Imaging, Department of Radiological Sciences.

Page 159:   Courtesy of Memorial Sloan-Kettering Cancer Center, New York.

Pages 160, 161:   Courtesy Stephen M. Pizer, Ph.D., and Henry Fuchs, Ph.D., Department of Computer Science, University of North Carolina, Chapel Hill, and Julian Rosenman, M.D., and George W. Scherouse, M.S., North Carolina Memorial Hospital.

Page 162:   Courtesy National Institutes of Health, Bethesda, Maryland.

Page 163:   Courtesy Stephen M. Pizer, Ph.D., Department of Computer Science, University of North Carolina, Chapel Hill.

Pages 164, 165:   Photo by Howard Sochurek taken in Department of Neurosurgery, University of Kansas Medical Center, Kansas City.

Page 166:   Courtesy of Gerald E. Schneider, Ph.D., Department of Brain and Cognitive Sciences, Massachusetts Institute of Technology, Cambridge.

Pages 168-169:   Courtesy Frederick P. Brooks, Jr., Ph.D., Department of Computer Science, University of North Carolina, Chapel Hill.

Pages 170-171:   Courtesy Department of Computer Science, University of North Carolina, Chapel Hill. GRIP molecular modelling project.

Page 173:   Photo by Howard Sochurek generated on Megavision 1024 XM System, Megavision Inc., Santa Barbara, California.

Page 174:   Courtesy University of Kansas Medical Center, Kansas City.

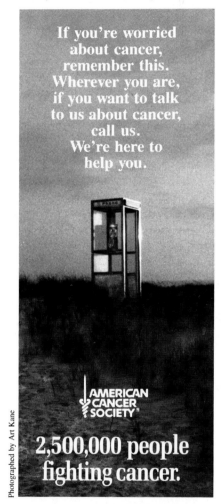

Photographed by Art Kane